PRAYER AS TRANSGRESSION?

ADVANCING STUDIES IN RELIGION

Series editor: Christine Mitchell

Advancing Studies in Religion catalyzes and provokes original research in the study of religion with a critical edge. The series advances the study of religion in method and theory, textual interpretation, theological studies, and the understanding of lived religious experience. Rooted in the long and diverse traditions of the study of religion in Canada, the series demonstrates awareness of the complex genealogy of religion as a category and as a discipline. ASR welcomes submissions from authors researching religion in varied contexts and with diverse methodologies.

The series is sponsored by the Canadian Corporation for Studies in Religion whose constituent societies include the Canadian Society of Biblical Studies, Canadian Society for the Study of Religion, Canadian Society of Patristic Studies, Canadian Theological Society, Société canadienne de théologie, and Société québécoise pour l'étude de la religion.

Prayer as Transgression?

The Social Relations of Prayer in Healthcare Settings

**SHERYL REIMER-KIRKHAM, SONYA SHARMA,
RACHEL BROWN, AND MELANIA CALESTANI**

with
Christina Beardsley, Lori G. Beaman, Paul Bramadat,
Sylvia Collins-Mayo, Andrew Todd, Christopher De Bono,
and Barry Quinn

McGill-Queen's University Press
Montreal & Kingston • London • Chicago

ISBN 978-0-2280-0164-5 (cloth)
ISBN 978-0-2280-0165-2 (paper)
ISBN 978-0-2280-0297-0 (ePDF)
ISBN 978-0-2280-0298-7 (ePUB)

Legal deposit third quarter 2020
Bibliothèque nationale du Québec

Printed in Canada on acid-free paper that is 100% ancient forest free
(100% post-consumer recycled), processed chlorine free.

This book has been published with the help of a grant from the Canadian Federation for the Humanities and Social Sciences, through the
Awards to Scholarly Publications Program, using funds provided by
the Social Sciences and Humanities Research Council of Canada.

Funded by the   Financé par le
Government   gouvernement   Canada Council   Conseil des arts
of Canada   du Canada   for the Arts   du Canada

We acknowledge the support of the Canada Council for the Arts.

Nous remercions le Conseil des arts du Canada de son soutien.

Library and Archives Canada Cataloguing in Publication

Title: Prayer as transgression? : the social relations of prayer in healthcare
    settings / Sheryl Reimer-Kirkham, Sonya Sharma, Rachel Brown, and
    Melania Calestani with Christina Beardsley, Lori Beaman, Paul Bramadat,
    Sylvia Collins-Mayo, Andrew Todd, Christopher De Bono, and Barry
    Quinn.
Names: Container of (work): Sharma, Sonya. Expressions of prayer in the
    everyday.
Series: Advancing studies in religion ; 9.
Description: Series statement: Advancing studies in religion ; 9 | Includes
    bibliographical references and index.
Identifiers: Canadiana (print) 20200269771 | Canadiana (ebook)
    20200270087 | ISBN 9780228001652 (paper) | ISBN 9780228001645 (cloth)
    | ISBN 9780228002970 (ePDF) | ISBN 9780228002987 (ePUB)
Subjects: LCSH: Health—Religious aspects—Christianity. | LCSH:
    Prayer—Christianity.
Classification: LCC BT732 .P73 2020 | DDC 261.8/321—dc23

This book was typeset by True to Type in 10.5/13 Sabon

Contents

Table and Figures

Preface

At the time we were writing this book, we, like many others, did not foresee a worldwide pandemic. This book project, and the research study it was based on, represents a BC ("before COVID-19") picture, but in many ways, what you will read was simply amplified during the time of the pandemic. More crisis, more constraints, more suffering, more innovation, more isolation, more prayer. The year 2020 saw substantial change in everyday life in personal and public dimensions, as the coronavirus raced and ravaged around the globe. Widespread job losses and economic hardships added to the generalized, societal angst that circulated as widely as the virus itself. Many were affected by the sudden death of a family member. The coronavirus was universalizing – no one was immune to it. At the same time, the impact on those populations who were structurally vulnerable was disproportionate; morbidity and mortality followed lines of social positioning, access to healthcare, and the strength of health systems (Quinn and Kumar 2014).

Given the book's focus, as researchers we asked each other, How are prayers being expressed? How do people do religion when they are asked to stay home because of social distancing and self-isolation? Google searches for "prayer" surged worldwide in step with the surge of emerging cases of COVID-19, according to Bentzen (2020), a European researcher. Government officials, such as Canada's Dr Theresa Tam, recognized the importance of religious observances such as Easter, Passover, Vaisakhi, and Ramadan for many citizens, asking them to assemble virtually via social media (Zimonjic 2020). Religious services online allowed people to participate from their living rooms, to try something they might have always been curious about or to commune virtually with others.

A paradox of the pandemic was the fast-moving nature of the disease alongside the slowing down of daily life to combat it. Staying at home, away from the physical places of work and school, caused difficult shifts in behaviour and routine for many. Yet it also meant reflection on the life taken for granted, with new appreciation for family, friends and neighbours, food procurement, observing, listening and being in nature, and exercise and creative pursuits. Life was lived on altered temporal terrains. Prayer was experienced through these activities that mirrored themes in our research: the lifting of spirit through the arts and nature, the comfort of ritual, prayer occurring in unexpected spaces, and the acts of kindness between people to help one another during an uncertain time. The self-isolation and social distancing meant religious rituals such as Friday Prayer, confession, and Holy Communion were lived out differently or stopped altogether. As a key theme of our book is transgression, praying in groups, serving each other bread and wine, or simply touching out of prayerful comfort would have crossed public health guidelines on limiting the contagion. Nonetheless, religion and spirituality continued to traverse public and private spaces. In addition to National Days of Prayer, people were encouraged to pray while they washed their hands. As the pandemic reached a crescendo, one Vancouver hospital was illuminated each night as a beacon of light to honour coming together in spirit, letting everyone know that they were not alone. Several countries showed their support of healthcare and key workers by leaning out of their windows or stepping onto their front doorsteps to clap their thanks for their work. It was a collective response that lifted spirits, a public moment expressed on the edges of private dwellings.

Hospitals are all at once public, chaotic, and intimate and where the pandemic was most keenly felt. They were where nurses and doctors at the point-of-care witnessed deep suffering and people dying without their loved ones near. Nurses and doctors picked up the emotional end-of-life care that might otherwise be offered by families and chaplains. Notwithstanding their profound knowledge and skill, there were many they could not save. They faced impossible choices, with accompanying moral distress that will carry forward for years. Staff were overwhelmed by demand, a shortage of personal protective equipment, and the worry of whether they carried the virus home to their families. Despite these concerns, some healthcare workers took time during their days to pray for each other and the sick (e.g.,

O'Kane 2020). Chaplains, part of healthcare provision, were barred from entering some hospitals by infectious disease precautions. Themselves social distancing by working from home, they adapted to this new reality by taking up "telechaplaincy" with indirect or technology-mediated support. They offered prayers and comfort over the phone to staff, patients, and families. Chaplains' liminality on the margins of healthcare services intensified because they were not visibly present, and yet, with the sweep of the virus, spiritual support was never more relevant nor sought after. Other healthcare organizations recognized this need and named chaplaincy as an "essential service," equipping them with personal protective equipment to do what they do best – bringing compassion and spiritual support to patients and staff in the darkest hours of the pandemic.

For many scholars, the pandemic prompted new queries about global relations, governance and economics, the environment, employment, housing, food security, and health and well-being. With regard to our project, the pandemic raised further questions about religion in the public sphere and more specifically the social relations of prayer in healthcare settings. We therefore invite our readers as you read this book to engage with these questions: What is different? What is similar? In light of the pandemic, how has prayer transgressed and transformed what was previously assumed about religion, spirituality and non-religion?

Acknowledgments

A book project such as this does not come about without the contributions of many. This book is a key outcome of a study named Prayer as Transgression? Exploring Accommodation of and Resistance to Prayer in Public Spaces, funded by Social Sciences and Humanities Research Council of Canada (SSHRC). We are grateful for generous funding that allowed us to conduct research in London and Vancouver, and meet as a team to discuss the project.

Thank you to the research sites. These healthcare organizations welcomed us and facilitated the many aspects of access required for such a project. We are indebted to the 109 participants who spoke with us and showed us the spaces in which prayer occurred. Their generosity, thoughtfulness, and enthusiasm for the study contribute to ongoing conversations about meaning and relationship in times of illness and crisis, social inclusion and equality, and religion in the public sphere. In London and Vancouver we also had the good fortune to hear from a diverse range of voices from across the healthcare system in the project's Practice Advisory Groups.

Our heartfelt thanks to our respective universities for research support in many forms, including research administrators and staff. At Trinity Western University's Research Office, we are thankful for assistance from Eve Stringham, vice-provost Research and Graduate Studies; and Sue Funk, research grants officer. At Kingston University London, we are thankful for assistance from Evanthia Lyons, head of the School of Law, Social and Behavioural Sciences; Emma Finch, research operations manager; and Agnieszka Wala, assistant accountant.

More practical but equally important, we are grateful to our research staff: Brenda Corcoran Smith (research coordinator), Christina

Beardsley (knowledge broker), Sandra Graham, Kyla Janzen, Anne Redmond, and Kelly Schutt (research assistants). We benefitted from your diligence with the hours you put into fieldwork and the inspiring analytic insights you brought to team discussions. Transcriptionists Jan Farquhar and Julene Reimer – we could not have done without your efficiency and commitment to help bring participants' stories into form. Thanks to Rebecca Kirkham for assistance with indexing. For those who contributed to the project through graphic design and social media platforms, you helped us to communicate what could be complex and ephemeral ideas: Ryan Schutt (website design), Helma Sawatzky (brochure design), Naomi Shields (report design), and Hannah Kirkham (photography).

Throughout the project we benefitted from interactions with academic colleagues and practitioners at various conferences and events, located at University of Toronto, University of Ottawa, University of Victoria, Simon Fraser University, Trinity Western University, Kingston University London, University of Lausanne, University of Leeds, Trinity College Dublin, University of Stirling, St George's University of London, the Association for the Sociology of Religion Conference in Seattle, Fraser Health Authority, and Vancouver Coastal Health.

Our sincere thanks to our publisher, McGill-Queen's University Press (MQUP), and in particular, Kyla Madden (senior editor) for her remarkable guidance in all aspects of preparing this manuscript, and to Ian MacKenzie (ParaGraphics) and Lisa Aitken (associate managing editor) for their attention to detail in the copy-editing process.

To our project team and co-authors for this book, we are profoundly grateful for the opportunity to have worked together. We came to this study from our own disciplines and backgrounds that greatly enriched our dialogues. The goodwill, intelligence, and laughter made for a most enjoyable research collaboration.

And to our partners, families, and friends, your interest in this project and your graciousness in supporting us during its tenure were invaluable and have meant the world to us.

Sheryl, Sonya, Rachel, and Melania

PRAYER AS TRANSGRESSION?

INTRODUCTION

Prayer as Transgression

Sheryl Reimer-Kirkham and Sonya Sharma

This book is about prayer, specifically prayer in hospitals. Prayer in hospitals provides a window onto religion in the public sphere. The question we pursue is, "What happens when prayer shows up in hospitals?" The research that informed this inquiry was framed with the questioning concept of "transgression" because of our interest to understand prayer as both welcome and unwelcome. In clinical contexts, prayer can be experienced as a counterpoint to the technologies, temporalities, and priorities of biomedicine. It can transgress or challenge unspoken social rules about a neutral, religion-free public space. Prayer can also trouble the distinctions made between religion and non-religion, and between the sacred and the profane. At other times, prayer can be unfamiliar, irrelevant, unwelcome, or inappropriate.

In this book we draw on a three-year critical ethnographic study that examined the social relations of prayer in hospitals, long-term care facilities, and community clinics in London and Vancouver. In these cities of remarkable religious diversity and social change, and in hospitals where this diverse "public" interacts in immediate and intimate ways, our study on prayer revealed how individuals, groups, and societies manage to work things out in the everyday. It is not that prayer is the main story, but rather prayer is a lens through which we examined this larger story. The social relations of prayer in healthcare settings turned out to tell us much about how people live well together, even in the face of personal crises and fragilities, social suffering, diversity, and social change.

More than one hundred pseudonymed participants[1] from twenty-one research sites in the two cities help to tell this story; they are peo-

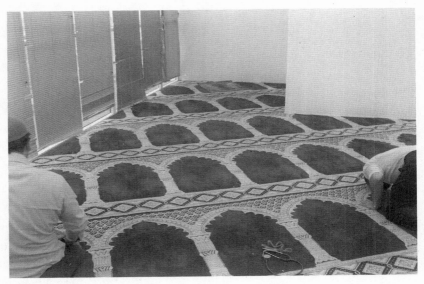

0.1 Muslim prayer room

ple who work in healthcare settings and people who have accessed healthcare services. Readers will be brought close to the lived realities of navigating diversity and how prayer can be a point of connection and conflict. As an example of prayer reaching across social differences, at one London hospital, Friday Prayer in the Muslim prayer room brought together patients and staff from various parts of the hospital, where hierarchies of position were put aside: "It's Friday Prayer, they need to pray, and they can't go somewhere else. The nearest [Muslim prayer room] is here and so they pop in, pray, and go. Anybody – clinical, non-clinical, patients – come in ... the helping, cooking, cleaning, all those departments" (Roshan, administrator, London) (see figure 0.1).

Ali, a Muslim chaplain,[2] described those who gathered for Friday Prayer at one London site: "On Friday's there are usually around 100–120 people attending the Friday Prayer: 60 per cent of the people attending the service are staff members. Then 10 per cent would be people from the local area, working maybe in local shops around the hospital. Thirty per cent would be visitors (family members) and patients, if able to move and attend. The nearest mosque is fifty minutes by bus from the hospital, so it is convenient for people around the hospital to come here." Prayer brought together people from the surrounding area from diverse social, ethnic, and class backgrounds. Mohamed, another London chaplain, said, "All people of all faiths pray [in the hospital]. ... Members and volunteers, visitors, everyone, patients, all of them commit the prayers there." As will be explained in chapter 3 on mapping geographies of prayer, the Muslim prayer room (a purpose-built space, which could accommodate more than 100 people – see figure 0.1) did not come about without conflict and negotiation, but the practice of prayer is now integrated into the day-to-day life of the clinical setting. This Muslim prayer room has brought a visibility of minority religion to the biomedical halls of the hospital and stands as testament to the state's Equality Act (2010), which requires accommodation of religious practices by England's public institutions, the National Health Service (NHS) included.

On the other side of the world, at a Vancouver hospital, we noted another way in which prayer reaches across biomedical and clinical differences. A patient was on his way to the surgical suite for cardiac surgery. It was 7 a.m., the surgeons were scrubbed and waiting for their first case of a busy day ahead. As the patient neared the pre-operative area, he interrupted the unfolding procedures, stating, "I can't go yet. I need to be prayed over. I need Frances [the chaplain]." The staff in the operating room called the chaplaincy office where "luckily another chaplain was already in. He can do it." Frances, who told this story, explained: "We take it very seriously if someone wants to pray before surgery. We take time." She took us to the stark pre-operative waiting area where this prayer occurred (see figure 0.2). She said she does not go home until she has checked whether there are pre-operative patients who might want prayer prior to their surgery the following day. She explained that in those cases "prayer travels with them" from their hospital room on the ward to the operating room. Thus prayer interrupts the clinical machinery of a world-leading cardiac program and enters the "staff only" spaces of the hospital. Prayer's forms in various clinical areas are analyzed in chapter 6.

In these two stories we observed prayer entering into the public institution of healthcare through the personal identities of individuals and collectives. Hospitals are porous to local constituencies and, more broadly, to the societal transformations that have come with migration and relocation. Hospitals become a landscape that is reconciling difficult histories and contemporary relations. The fact that

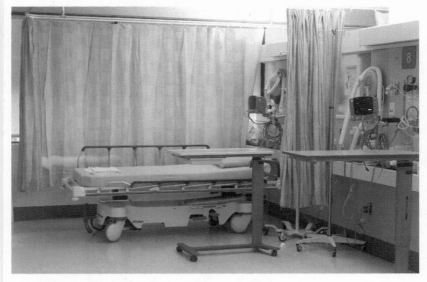

o.2 Pre-operative room where patients wait for surgery

hospitals do so in the face of human suffering, unpredictability and crisis, intimacy and immediacy means these social trends are amplified and more visible and require even more urgent responses.

Expressions of prayer were attuned to and shaped by the suffering experienced in hospitals and could be understood to enter into and transgress the highly technical, fast-paced, disease-oriented, curative, and complex cultures of clinical settings. Mark (administrator, Vancouver) reflected on the disjuncture between clinical care and spirituality, and the transgressive presence of spirituality and prayer: "Hospitals, by nature, are very scientific places. They're full of smart people who've been trained in their discipline of science. So you juxtapose that with a topic of spirituality [and prayer] and you're in two different worlds ... it's transgressive." Generally speaking, both in the administrative structures of healthcare and in the education of healthcare professionals, religion plays a minimal role, such that religiously informed values, beliefs, and practices that relate to health and illness experiences are often neglected. This contrast of "two different worlds" maps onto the distinction anthropologist Arthur Kleinman (1988) makes between disease and illness; between the biomedical model and the biopsychosocial model. Oriented toward disease as only an alteration in biological structure or functioning, clinical care is focused on cure. In the biopsychosocial model, illness is understood as "the embodiment of the symbolic network linking body, self, and society" (Kleinman 1988, 6). In the narratives of this book are examples of where prayer could bridge constructions of disease and illness, to create meaning and healing in the midst of biomedicine's focus on curing the body. To the extent that the limits of biomedicine are becoming more apparent and healthcare professions are more open to consider the place of patient spirituality within the experience of illness (Balboni and Peteet 2017), space is opening for deeper engagement with the intersections of religion and spirituality, health and well-being, illness and suffering.

Anthropologist Veena Das (2015) writes about suffering as sometimes ordinary and chronic, other times catastrophic and crisis-laden. When suffering is understood in these ways, it encompasses the multifaceted social suffering that results from what political, economic, and institutional power does to people, and how these forms of power themselves influence responses to social problems (Kleinman, Das, and Lock 1997). Such an expanded interpretation of social suffering aligns with anthropologist Henrik Vigh's (2008) extension of the meanings attributed to crisis. He explains that crisis (especially in high-resource countries) is constructed as a singular event – "an intermediary moment of chaos" – that ruptures the order of things; yet for a great many people around the world, crisis is endemic (i.e., crisis *as* context) rather than episodic (i.e., crisis *in* context). With the social relations of prayer as our project's centre, we have tuned to prayer in relation to social suffering and chronic crisis. We have come to understand how rituals in a city park to remember those who have died unexpectedly during Vancouver's opioid crisis (see chapter 6) are naming the social suffering of lives marked by chronic crisis. How for persons with dementia who are institutionalized, prayer can serve as a reminder of their personhood and thereby disrupt what could be viewed as a state of chronic crisis. How staff, who may themselves face precarious circumstances in the midst of austerity measures in the NHS or uncertain citizenship after the Brexit vote, visit a chapel at lunchtime to write a prayer for employment in a prayer book. How an Indigenous[3] elder, even though she is treated rudely by staff, remains resolute in offering healing ceremony to a hospitalized community member and thereby experiences and mitigates social suffering.

ON PRAYER AND TRANSGRESSION

Prayer shows up in hospitals in a variety of forms, circumstances, and places (see chapter 1). In diverse hospital settings, where people from all walks of life cross paths, prayer can emerge in unlikely ways and spaces. The above exemplar, of the patient who requested prayer before surgery could proceed, demonstrated the crossing of the sacred into the seemingly secular space of biomedicine. Another example was of chaplains and healthcare staff from religious and spiritually diverse backgrounds coming together for prayer for a patient who had recently died. The building of a Muslim prayer room in a social context that has experienced simultaneously the decline of Christianity, the rise of no religion, and a more religiously diverse society is another example of the variation of prayer at work.

Prayer is described as the heart of religion; in the words of philosopher and psychologist William James, "Prayer is the very soul and essence of religion.... [P]rayer is religion in act" (James 1902, as quoted in Mason 2013, 24). Sociologist Michael Mason states, "Far from being just one religious practice among others, prayer is the believer's 'respiration,' the most vital activity upon which all others depend. It makes the sacred real" (9). Prayer is an ancient practice and like other spiritual concepts is difficult to define. Although there is some disciplinary variance, the general understanding is that prayer involves connection between humans and the divine (Bender 2008). For the participants in our study, such an interpretation of prayer was most common, though there was much variation in the forms of theistic prayer.

However, meanings of prayer extended well beyond those associated with institutional religion, with "the believer," or even the "divine." For example, we observed that for the non-religious, prayer may connote a moment of silence. Prayer may take form in a non-theistic ritual in response to loss or grief. In the First Nations sacred space at a downtown Vancouver hospital, prayer involved the Indigenous tradition of smudging. On a psychiatric unit, art therapy for some was understood as prayer. We delve into diverse expressions of prayer in chapter 1, and the materiality of prayer in chapter 8. How is it that these diverse practices could all be interpreted as prayer? The question is particularly germane in Canada's and England's increasingly non-religious societies. Linda Woodhead, a sociologist of religion, suggests the helpful idea of prayer as "changing the subject": "prayer as switching the conversation in one's head, taking a new subject-position or viewpoint (including God's), moving to a new emotional register, altering focus, or dissociating from one state and entering another 'higher' one" (2015b, 213). She continues, "Contemporary prayer ... is a personally-meaningful experience with a close relation to an individual's own life concerns, hopes and fears" (233). Prayer thus externalizes the concerns of the person or people who pray. Our participants illustrated this externalizing as prayer in that there was a transcending of the self. Such an understanding of prayer begins to create space for less-scripted and non-religious forms of prayer, along with the formalized and religious. Moreover, prayer is somehow special or "set apart" and transcends or goes beyond a moment or situation. Although prayer took various forms, the shared participant view was of prayer as distinctive from other spiritual and non-spiritual actions. Many viewed prayer as communing with God or a higher power, but prayer was also viewed as transcending present circumstances through a sense of the mystical, or an experience of deep understanding or profound relational connection (Reimer-Kirkham, Sharma, and Corcoran Smith 2019, 2).

The framing of the study with the question "Prayer as transgression?" raised various responses as we introduced the project to participants, including, "Prayer is not negative," or, "I don't agree that prayer is a transgression." Several people associated the word *transgression* with the Lord's Prayer from the Christian tradition, where one asks the Lord for forgiveness for one's trespasses (i.e., transgressions) just as one is requested to forgive those who have trespassed against one. Such responses were not entirely surprising, given that religions can seem concerned predominantly with controlling and eliminating transgression, as anthropologist Michael Taussig notes (1998). Yet if we look at prayer as transgression from another angle, we can see other possibilities (Sharma, Reimer-Kirkham, and Cochrane 2013). As Jane, a Vancouver chaplain, put it, "When I pray with people, they pray with me, we are crossing boundaries. It's not like anything else because prayer crosses so much. It crosses people's lives. It crosses faith traditions." This quote illustrates the draw toward expansive interpretations of prayer and transgression. Thus we needed conceptual limits of these terms. We come to a definition of transgression through feminist and social theorists who view transgression as the ability to go beyond limits and conventions, to deny and affirm differences, to move against and beyond boundaries (e.g., hooks 1994; Taussig 1998).

Hence we were interested in how the sacred (with religious and non-religious meanings) might disrupt the order of things, including clinical contexts. We wanted to know how prayer could potentially shift the seemingly rational and secular nature of healthcare. French philosopher and social theorist Michel Foucault explained that limit and transgression depend on each other and that "a limit could not exist if it was absolutely uncrossable, and, reciprocally, transgression would be pointless if it merely crossed a limit composed of illusions and shadows" (Foucault 1977 in Carrette 1999, 60). Foucault was curious about what becomes of a limit after a transgression, the moment that limits do not contain. Our study on prayer aimed to attend to the limits that prevented prayer from happening, but also the limits that prayer transgressed and transformed, altering lived experiences and clinical contexts and temporalities.

From our research, in brief, we learned that:

- Prayer transgressed any assumption of a religion-free (entirely secular) public space.
- Prayer transgressed social difference such as that created by structures of race, gender, and class. In some cases, perceptions of difference were diminished by prayer; in other cases, difference was amplified.
- Prayer transgressed the concerns that mark healthcare settings, to open spaces in which to experience, relate, think differently, and contemplate the metaphysical (Reimer-Kirkham, Sharma, and Corcoran Smith 2019, 3).

Transgression applied to prayer could, therefore, be viewed as negative and positive to the extent that it could interrupt, transform, and reinforce. By employing the lens of transgression, we have been able to "trouble" prayer by examining the social relations of prayer at the micro, meso, and macro levels, considering how religion is used toward certain ends, and uncovering how prayer can serve inclusionary and exclusionary purposes. We heed urban theorist Renata Hejduk's contention that transgression "breaks through the everyday or profane and allows questioning of boundaries, systems and ideal constructions moving into a more fluid and pressing space" of social relations and the sacred (2010, 280). This heuristic contribution of the concept of transgression can be understood, as Taussig (1998) puts it, as reading backwards as well as forwards to see the interplay of sacred and sacrilege. In the chapters that follow, transgression is applied as an analytic tool to understand the social relations of prayer in the diverse landscape of public healthcare.

ON TENSIONS AND THEORY

The provocative question "Prayer as transgression?" prompted reflexivity for us as researchers. The question helped to identify norms and standards we easily slipped into, such as assuming that prayer is generally a good activity to engage in, that prayer is commonplace, or that prayer can be stretched to encompass an array of spiritual practices. We found ourselves navigating several interrelated tensions common to research on religion in our contemporary era.

Definitional and Political Tensions

We are cautious about the prevalent dichotomy between religion and spirituality in health literature (in particular) whereby religion is considered as political, often harmful, and institutionalized, and spirituality is considered as neutral, life-affirming, and personally meaningful (Bramadat, Coward, and Stajduhar 2013). In our study, some participants identified strongly with spirituality but not at all with religion, others identified more with religion and to some extent with spirituality, and yet others were ambivalent about or antagonistic to both terms. To capture such varying perceptions, we hold to the following conceptualizations of religion and spirituality: Religion is difficult to define in any universalist sense but carries transcendent (sacred) and social dimensions, with the practice of it often occurring through relatively formal social institutions. Spirituality, while also having to do with the metaphysical, has been interpreted as less institutionalized and as a more individual expression of values and beliefs but nonetheless grounded in material concerns and relations of power (Bramadat, Coward, and Stajduhar 2013; Henery 2003). Non-religion involves meaning systems that are typically non-theist but may or may not have transcendent, metaphysical, or existential referents or effects (e.g., wonder and awe).

Constructs such as the sacred and the divine have been employed to anchor definitions of religion and spirituality and to thereby distinguish these from other phenomena such as culture or society. Following from sociologist Émile Durkheim ([1915] 2008) and historian

Mircea Eliade ([1959] 1987), properties of the sacred are typically contrasted to the profane. Broadly stated, the sacred, as extraordinary and beyond individual creation, stands apart from the profane as ordinary and part of everyday life. However, deciding what might be deemed as "standing apart" continues as a core problematic for scholars of religion, especially when considering its relationship to secularity, secularism, and various forms of non-religion (Lee 2015; Taves 2009). Here the typology of psychologist Ann Taves is helpful in anchoring broader interpretations of the sacred. She constructs "continua of specialness ranging from the ordinary to the very special with some things considered so special that they are set apart and protected by taboos" (44). Things set apart can involve spiritual beings (e.g., deities); absolutes or ideal things (e.g., values); mystical or spiritual qualities of places, objects, experiences; or events that are in themselves without agency. In our study, prayer transgressed the ordinary and the set apart, the profane and the sacred, with a range of prayer experiences described by participants as special or set apart.

Another set of tensions relate to the nature of prayer itself and the degree to which it is an individual act or a social act. There is a tendency, especially in the West, to view prayer as a personal and private practice. And yet, as is also revealed in our study, prayer shapes and is shaped by power relations and social structures. Sociologist of religion Robert Orsi states, "Prayer is a good example of a religious practice that is misidentified as private and so therefore assumed not to have a history or a politics. But people at prayer are intimately engaged and implicated in their social worlds – prayer is a switching point between the social world and the imagination" (2003, 173). Prayer can be a personal conversation that one has with God, but it is also embedded in and influenced by social life.

Our framing of transgression prompted us to interrogate the assumption that politics and religion operate as separate categories, as in the notion that healthcare as a secular space is non-religious. As a publicly funded part of the government apparatus, healthcare could be understood as an arena differentiated and emancipated from religious institutions and norms (Casanova 1994). Public institutions are sites where the secularization of modernity has by and large resulted in institutions that no longer need or are interested in maintaining a "sacred cosmos or maintaining a public religious worldview" (Taylor 2007, 37). Yet modernity does not imply "a reduction in the level of religious belief or practice or that religion is necessarily relegated to a private sphere." Rather, as sociologist José Casanova contends, "it is not only to discover but to affirm a legitimate public role for religion in the modern world" (Casanova 1994, as quoted in Davie 2013, 51). Thus secularization as we understand it is linked to modernity playing an active role in structuring the expression of the secular and the non-secular. Hospitals are spaces in which one can observe this intersection and its transformation.

Intermingled with these definitional and political tensions was an ever-present challenge to hold space for the non-religious – who might or might not pray – and for those who saw prayer as irrelevant, unfamiliar, or unwelcome. While prayer may indeed be expansive, even among nones,[4] as noted by sociologist Elizabeth Drescher (2016), there is a lack of knowledge about the rapidly growing sector of Canadians and Britons who are non-religious, unaffiliated, or not committed (Bullock 2017; Lee 2015; Wilkins-Laflamme 2017b). Revealed in our study (and described in more detail later in this Introduction, chapter 2, chapter 7, and appendix 1) were a complex mix of identities that challenged any assumptions about who might or might not pray. A common underlying supposition in much of healthcare literature on spirituality and chaplaincy is that people are by nature spiritual and therefore might well be amenable to prayer (Hudson 2012). This subtle universalism is at play in our data. Our task as analysts has been, for example, to not impose an interpretation of prayer onto practices such as yoga, ritual, and meditation where participants might not view them as prayer.

Guiding Theoretical Frameworks

To keep these tensions with their associated relations of power in our conscious frames of reference, we have drawn on the interrelated theoretical traditions of lived religion, intersectionality, and deep equality. Sociologist Meredith McGuire explains that "religion as lived" captures "how religion and spirituality are practised, experienced and expressed by ordinary people (rather than official spokespersons) in the context of their everyday lives" (2008, 15, 12). Orsi states, "[Lived] religion is situated amid the ordinary concerns of life, at the junctures of self and culture, family and social world.… [R]eligion is always religion-in-action, religion-in-relationships between people" (2003, 172; also see Ammerman 2007; Bender 2003). Religion and therefore prayer are experienced as woven into people's day-to-day lives such as work, leisure, education, and family. The theoretical concept of lived religion allowed us to study the everyday occurrences of prayer in clinical settings and how they were entwined with relations of power embedded in the social and biomedical worlds of hospitals, street clinics, and long-term care facilities.

Intersectionality, with its roots in feminism, post-colonialism, and critical race theory, has not been as widely taken up in religious studies (Davis and Zarkov 2017; Reimer-Kirkham and Sharma 2011; Weber 2015) but nonetheless offers considerable analytic advantage to our study on prayer in healthcare. Intersectionality focuses on "how social structures make certain identities the consequence of and the vehicle for vulnerability" (Crenshaw 2016), such that some people and not others face exclusion. Social, institutional, and individual processes can enable and challenge social inequalities experienced by those of faith and of none. With intersectional attention to the social structures that lead to advantage and disadvantage, assumptions about religion and related social relations of power are scrutinized in order to make visible religion as a social phenomenon in daily life and offer a social critique of hegemonic religion and its potential misuse (Bilge 2010; Mirza 2013; Sharma and Lewellyn 2016; Wilkins 2008). Intersectionality guided us to look behind the preponderance of chaplains who self-identify as Christian, as symbolic of the subtle but ongoing hegemonic presence of majoritarian religion in these hospitals in London and Vancouver (models of chaplaincy are described in chapter 5). The theoretical framing of intersectionality has also allowed us to interrogate colonial residues in both sites, where, for example, Indigenous peoples continue to suffer the legacies of religiously affiliated residential schools, and where racialized diaspora from British colonies are visible in their spiritual practices of prayer while at the same time their services are subtly framed as marginal.

Also influenced by critical social theories, including feminist theory, the recent theory of deep equality, developed by sociologist Lori G. Beaman (2014, 2017a), shifts our primary angle of analysis to those responses to relations of power that hint at how differences are negotiated in positive ways. Deep equality tunes not to difference on the one hand, or sameness on the other hand, but rather to reconciliatory middle ground in similarities. Quoting Beaman (2017a, 13), "Deep equality is not a legal, policy, or social prescription, nor is it achievable by a magic formula that can be enshrined in human rights codes.... [I]t relocates equality as a process rather than a definition, and as lived rather than prescribed." By orienting toward the everyday negotiation of religious diversity by ordinary people, rather than legally bound concerns of accommodation and tolerance, the lens of deep equality allowed us to work across micro, meso, and macro levels to see how agonistic respect at every level could create conditions for living well together. Everyday occurrences of prayer in the face of the vulnerabilities and intimacies associated with illness and hospitals have provided new insights into how deep equality can be achieved (see chapter 2).

THE RESEARCH CONTEXTS

Why did we select Vancouver and London as research contexts? These cities serve as two interesting case studies, with similarities and differences. Both are in countries with public healthcare systems. They are expensive cities, and that affects how social inequalities show up and are worked out in healthcare systems. Vancouver and London are located in countries with widening wealth gaps. Both cities are linked through histories of colonialism and empire. And both reflect superdiversity (Vertotec 2007), with high levels of religious and ethnic diversity, including growing populations that identify with no religion.

In Canada, immigration from Asia, the Middle East, and Africa has created ever-growing Buddhist, Hindu, Muslim, and Sikh communities (7.2 per cent of Canada's population; Statistics Canada 2011). At the same time, increasing numbers of Canadians (24 per cent) and Britons (25 per cent) are indicating "no religion" on census surveys (Statistics Canada 2011; ONS 2012). Indigenous peoples comprise 4.9 per cent of the population in Canada (Statistics Canada 2017a) and are diverse in their tribal identities and religious affiliations. Following centuries of land dispossession and colonial oppressions, many of which were operationalized by the church through residential schools that "were part of a process that brought European states and Christian churches together in a complex and powerful manner" (TRC 2015, 43), Indigenous peoples have an uneasy relationship with organized religion and are focused on restoring traditional spiritual practices while calling all Canadians to engage in reconciliation.

According to the 2011 census, England's current religious profile shows 59 per cent self-identifying as Christian, 25 per cent as nones, 5 per cent as Muslim, 4 per cent adhering to religions including (in order of frequency) Hinduism, Sikhism, Buddhism, and Judaism, and another 7 per cent who do not indicate religion (i.e., missing data) (ONS 2012). More recently, the British Social Attitudes Survey reported that 52 per cent of people in Britain now identify as belonging to no religion (Curtice et al. 2019). These trends are heightened in the context of healthcare, where the fragility of life intersects with a range of values and beliefs, faith traditions and rituals, including prayer.

Both Vancouver and London differ from respective national averages in significant ways. Vancouver is located in Cascadia, the region from California to British Columbia (sometimes referred to as the Pacific Northwest). Those who identify as Christian comprise less than half of Vancouver's population (41.7 per cent; compared to Canada's 67 per cent; Statistics Canada 2011), with an equal number who identify as "no religion" (41.5 per cent; compared to Canada's 24 per cent; Statistics Canada 2011). Cascadia has been characterized by a "live and let live" attitude; ecological spiritualities with deep connections to the landscape and environment; a diversity of individualized, eclectic spiritualities; and a strong social ethic. Christianity has historically had less influence in structuring society in this region, as there has not been a state church or a dominant Christian majoritarian religious centre as in other parts of Canada (Wilkins-Laflamme, 2017b). This region also has higher levels of immigration (41 per cent of Vancouverites are foreign born, compared to Canada's 22 per cent; Statistics Canada 2017b), with over 15 per cent of citizens reporting as Sikh, Buddhist, Muslim, or Hindu (in order of frequency; compared to Canada's 7.2 per cent; Statistics Canada 2011). The influence on prayer of ecological spiritualities in Vancouver, and London's arts and culture scene are picked up in chapter 9.

Theologian and sociologist of religion Stephen Bullivant (2017, 3) states that according to the European Social Survey (2014) and British Social Attitudes Survey (2015), London "has by far, the fewest Nones in Britain at 31% (compared to 58% in the South East, and 56% in Scotland). Inner London also has, by far, the highest proportion of those from Non-Christian religions (28%)." Members of minority religious traditions have grown. This is seen in the high proportion of Muslims (12.4 per cent) (ONS 2012) and the rise of black majority churches (i.e., Pentecostal and evangelical traditions) in London between 2005 and 2012 (Brierley 2013). In the midst of religious change, rising social inequalities are evident, levels of debt are increasing to cover basic household costs, and the provision of a social net provided by government welfare has become precarious. This precarity has meant faith groups, organizations, and institutions are extending and resuming their duties, stepping in where the state cannot (Bäckström et al. 2016).

With regard to prayer, a 2015 Angus Reid poll (Angus Reid Institute 2016) reported that 86 per cent of Canadians had prayed in the past year. These numbers would (at a basic read) suggest that prayer occurs for those who are religious and non-religious. Yet in British Columbia, with its higher proportion of nones, 51 per cent of the population in 2014 responded that they never practice lone religious or spiritual activities, such as prayer or meditation (Wilkins-Laflamme 2017a). In Britain, six out of seven believed that prayers can be answered or "believe in prayer" (Bingham 2013), and 25 per cent of nones said they pray, some as often as daily (Bullivant 2017). Religious historian Clive Field draws on several reports and surveys to state that in Britain, "self-reported regular (weekly or more) private prayer has declined from one-half to one-quarter of the population over the past century" (2017, 92). The picture, thus, is one of continued belief in prayer, though the actual practice of prayer has declined significantly.

With this degree of diversity and social change, the question follows as to how Canada and England regulate religion. In Canada, the Charter of Human Rights and Freedom (1982) and the Multiculturalism Act (1988) form the legislative framework. The charter provides that every individual is equal before and under the law and has the right to equal benefit without discrimination based on, in particular, race, national or ethnic origin, colour, religion, sex, age, or mental or physical disability. In England, the Equality Act 2010 brings together separate pieces of legislation into one single Act. This Act provides a legal framework to protect the rights of individuals and to promote an equal society. It legislates for the protection of age, disability, gender reassignment, marriage and civil partnership, pregnancy and maternity, race, religion or belief, sex, and sexual orientation (Equality and Human Rights Commission 2017). Though equality and human rights are legislated by these Acts, these legislative frameworks in both Canada and England more often operate to the goals of accommodation and tolerance. Beaman (2012, 2017a) points out that the language of accommodation implies that privileged groups can "give" accommodation to a lesser group, thus creating an inherent inequality.

THE STUDY

To get at the social relations of prayer, we conducted fieldwork in twenty-one hospitals, clinics, and long-term care facilities in Vancouver and London (funded by the Social Sciences and Humanities Research Council #435-2015-1729). The research sites were alike as publicly funded healthcare organizations, but also varied in some important ways, including that some sites were religiously affiliated. In our research, this was when a faith community contributed closely to shaping and administering a healthcare setting. These similarities and differences are further described in chapter 4 in an examination of organizational practices in the management of prayer. We underwent ethical review for the project at these sites, as well as at a Canadian and a British university.

Fieldwork involved talking, walking, listening, observing, writing, and absorbing. We interviewed chaplains as our entrée to the project. They took us to various places in their facilities where meaningful prayer encounters had occurred and told us about them. They also wrote reflections in research diaries. In addition, we interviewed administrators, healthcare professionals (e.g., doctors, nurses, social workers), and spiritual care volunteers, including community faith leaders. We also spoke with former patients and families about their views on prayer in hospitals. These varied sources of data were carefully analyzed through a team process that involved line-by-line coding, followed by categorization of the codes we developed, and finally thematic analysis, which resulted in the topics we present in this book (see detailed description in appendices 1 and 2).

Prayer encompasses much. To study it solely from theological, anthropological, social, or health outcomes perspectives seemed incomplete in healthcare settings. Rather, we saw the value of bringing together an interdisciplinary team to study prayer from various disciplinary vantage points and social locations. Many of us were already working across disciplinary lines, which meant we could draw from expertise in health studies (Brenda Corcoran Smith, Barry Quinn, and Sheryl Reimer-Kirkham), sociology (Lori G. Beaman, Sylvia Collins-Mayo, and Sonya Sharma), religious studies (Paul Bramadat and Rachel Brown), anthropology (Melania Calestani), and theology and chaplaincy studies (Christina Beardsley, Christopher De Bono, and Andrew Todd). We are at different points in our careers, both practitioners and academics, and of various ethnic heritages and gender identities. Our team was located in Vancouver and London and represented a variety of religious and non-religious affiliations, which in itself drew us into reflexive positions as we listened to each other and thought deeply about what shaped us and the phenomena we were investigating. Our national differences meant we were in a constant ethnographic mode, as we visited each other's sites, mused what a national spirituality might look like, and considered respective cultural imaginaries: nature and ecologies in Vancouver, the arts and culture in London; coffee for the Canucks, tea for the Brits.

Project leads, nurse scholar Sheryl Reimer-Kirkham and sociologist Sonya Sharma, worked closely with a core team (Christina Beardsley, Rachel Brown, Melania Calestani, and Brenda Corcoran Smith) to collect and analyze the data. The project leads and core team took leadership on the book chapters, with invaluable contributions from co-investigators and collaborators (Lori G. Beaman, Paul Bramadat, Sylvia Collins-Mayo, Christopher De Bono, Barry Quinn, and Andrew Todd). We discussed our ideas at length at an initial think tank with the London contributors (March 2017) and again at a think tank in Vancouver with both London and Vancouver contributors (September 2017). Authorship of chapters was decided on the basis of people's interests and with chapter contributors representing both research sites. Because of the cohesive process of envisioning the project, conducting fieldwork, working with a large data set, and writing collaboratively – all the while benefitting tremendously from our respective areas of expertise – we ask the reader to read this as a coherent story about prayer in hospitals, and what it tells us about religion in the public sphere.

Expressions of Prayer in the Everyday

Sonya Sharma and Sheryl Reimer-Kirkham

A research diary excerpt: One of the nurses who is Buddhist is quite insistent that I bless rooms after a resident has died and before the next resident moves in. She believes the spirits need permission and assistance to leave. She knows that I am Christian and is happy for whatever type of prayer I wish to offer. This has become our ritual, not something expected by or known about among other staff members.

This informal ritual recently became more public. A resident died one evening and prior to the body being picked up by the funeral home three separate staff members heard a noise from the room that sounded like the resident's very distinct form of calling out for help. They entered the room to check, confirmed that the resident was indeed dead, but were left unsettled by the experience. The story spread among the staff. When the nurse arrived in the morning she phoned me immediately and asked me to come pray for the room as a new resident would be arriving within the hour.

I found the nurse and several staff members waiting for me. Among the staff gathered there was a Roman Catholic, a Christian, a Hindu, someone "spiritual but not religious," our Buddhist nurse and me. We all agreed on a blessing so that the room would be a place of peace and comfort. I prayed for the person who had died, for her family, for the new person about to arrive and for the care team who say "good-bye" and then "hello" so frequently and so quickly. The group appeared satisfied and expressed appreciation. We then went about the rest of our day.

Annalise, chaplain, Vancouver

As noted in the Introduction to this book, our research came across many expressions of prayer, and there is much about prayer in this excerpt from Annalise's research diary. It shows the form that prayer took, expressing it verbally and standing among a group of colleagues. Annalise described the process of how the prayer came about: the death of a resident and the response of the staff to it, resulting in their gathering to pray. She also told about its substance – to bless and release the room of spirits; and its function – to prepare the room for the next resident and to put the staff at ease. This experience of prayer was also evidence of the social relations of prayer between people who had varied orientations to prayer but agreed on the intention of prayer and, despite their diverse backgrounds, shared a common belief, even though they may call or construct it differently.

In this chapter, we reflect on expressions of prayer in Vancouver and London healthcare settings as a frame with which to engage the following chapters of this book. First, we address the meaning of prayer itself, moving between how prayer has been theorized by sociologists, psychologists, and religionists, and how prayer was described by our participants, with rich data revealing diverse forms of prayer. Second, we show how prayer was enacted by considering four overlapping areas that tend to be included in taxonomies of prayer (e.g., ap Sion 2015; Geertz 2016), and that similarly emerged in our analysis: *form*, the various modes prayers took; *substance*, the content included in prayers; *process*, the ways in which prayers came about; and *function*, the use or application of prayer.

ON MEANINGS OF PRAYER

Many scholars have attempted to understand what prayer is. Anthropologist and sociologist Marcel Mauss (2003) explained that prayer is a religious and oral act that enables relationship to the sacred. In Annelise's narrative, the sacred is constructed as the metaphysical, a space that has to do with spirits and the divine. Others have unlinked prayer from religious and sacred associations (Drescher 2016). Importantly, prayer is shaped by the social and cultural contexts in which it occurs. Even though prayer may happen when one is alone, it is never enacted without some connection to the social relations in which it is situated and existing cultural norms (Giordan 2015). In our research, four coinciding aspects were consistent in participants' descriptions and understandings of the meaningfulness of prayer. They were relational, distinctive, emotional, and political (e.g., Mason 2015; Mauss 2003; Taves 2009; van der Veer 2016).

Prayer as Relational

The commonplace understanding of prayer involves a connection between humans and the divine or another being or energy life force, and can be shared among and between those religious and non-religious. It can also be considered an approach (or not) to mindfulness, meditation, and personal meaningfulness that emphasizes the inner world of the individual in relation to the external (see Giordan and Woodhead 2013, 2015). In the responses to our question of how participants understood prayer, we found a spectrum of interpretations within the broad catchment of prayer as "connecting with the sacred." At one end of this spectrum were those who held religiously embedded views, where prayer was communication with God. Some used succinct phrases such as "communing with God," reflecting both intimate ("communing") and transcendent ("with God") dimensions. The relational aspect between the one praying and the one prayed to was emphasized by many, with the following example from a citizen in London: "It's about communication and listening and hearing what God says." At the other end of the spectrum were those who held nontheistic views, where prayer might involve deeper insight into self or connection to nature (see chapter 9). Martin described prayer as a form of consciousness: "My understanding of prayer is that it's the internal experience and people will pay attention to their internal experience or not" (chaplain, London). In the middle of the spectrum were interpretations that involved transcendence of the everyday, but not limited to God, Yahweh, or Allah. Curtis said, "Prayer transcends the reality around by its very nature, it is connecting with that which is beyond" (chaplain, Vancouver). Regardless of potential partners in prayer, respondents referred to these entities as actors who can hear, understand, and respond to their requests (Cerulo and Barra 2008, 378). It seems that Annalise and the staff, in their intentionality of this room-blessing ritual, were praying with the expectation that they were heard. Andreas summed up this spectrum in his understanding of prayer: "Prayer is how we connect with a superior being, deity, or just our own deeper self" (chaplain, Vancouver).

Prayer as Distinctive

Psychologist Ann Taves (2009) suggests that the domain of the sacred be understood as what is special or set apart. In her work on prayer among the non-religious, sociologist Elizabeth Drescher (2016, 163) found that prayer was discursively and experientially distinctive from other spiritual or non-spiritual actions. These interpretations resonate with our data in which prayer was constructed by our participants as special, either by its referent (i.e., God, deity, higher power, or non-empirical other) or by its association (i.e., with what is special or set apart). The distinctiveness of prayer as perceived by those in our study involved a sense of awe. Andreas said, "Prayer is a way to be in the world allowing the mystical to take place, and not having all the questions answered." The specialness of prayer was reflected in how cautious participants were to not enter into it lightly or without permission. Its specialness was also evidenced when some teared up during our conversations about prayer, or when they told us that they had spent much time thinking about our research project. Annalise, for example, said she decided to remain in her chaplaincy post because thinking about prayer encounters with residents, patients, and families in the context of our project made her realize how she valued her role and how special such encounters were.

Prayer in healthcare settings and in times of illness and crisis could all the more be set apart, with participants describing situations of deep searching and meaning-making. Kirstie, a citizen in London who experienced time in hospital, said, "I remember receiving communion at the bedside from the chaplain when I wasn't able to get to the chapel. That was very important and meaningful." On the one hand, her illness and receiving prayer at the bedside marked this moment as extraordinary. On the other hand, for Kirstie, prayer could be experienced as special during the mundane tasks of everyday life: "It's feeling the presence of God when you're doing the washing up." In the case of the room-blessing in the opening scenario, the perceived urgency with which the prayer came about – "she phoned me immediately" – signals that what is about to take place is distinct and set apart, even though the transition of patients through a clinical space or long-term care room is a routine event. Prayer can take place in varied contexts but be simultaneously distinct.

Prayer as Emotional

In the descriptions of prayer given above, the emotional presence is obvious. Words used to describe prayer such as *peace, comfort, encouraging,* or *deep meaning* reflect the emotion worlds present in the giving and receiving of prayer. Similarly, in Annalise's narrative of the room blessing, words of *unsettled, satisfied,* and *appreciation* communicate emotion. Just as prayer is sociologically understood as intersubjective and relational, so are emotions, viewed as "constituted in the relations between people" (Lupton 1998, 6). Emotion in prayer articulates "a wide range of thoughts and feelings operating at various levels of awareness" (Miller and Stiver 1997, 143). Shannon, a healthcare professional in London, told us, "I do pray with people and it's very much a heartfelt sentiment from whatever it is that people are feeling." Sociologist Arlie Hochschild (2003, 17) states that "emotion communicates information." It communicates feedback through the body, which can be linked to the intersubjectivity that has been described in prayer experiences between staff (chaplains, administrators, and healthcare professionals), patients, and family members.

In this book the focus is on the social relations of prayer, which means rational and cognitive understandings of prayer are not foregrounded. Indeed, some participants did think of prayer as "neurophysiological" or "rational," but this was not a strong theme to emerge from our data. Similarly, doctrinal understandings such as "Prayer as a gift from God to us" did not feature as a prominent theme, perhaps because of the research setting of healthcare, where life is often experienced as intimate and fragile and encompassing a range of emotional responses. Instead of posing a rational/emotion binary on understandings of prayer, we look to feminist scholars (Game 1997; Jagger 1989) who have argued for mutually constitutive conceptualizations between knowledge and emotion, mind and body. Emotion is a way of knowing the world, and knowing the world is not based simply on cognition or intellect. Thus both are required in the understanding of expressions of prayer. For example, Chiara (citizen, London) stated, "What is a prayer? It is an externalization of a feeling and a request." Prayer is an expression of both emotion and knowledge. Tulio (chaplain, Vancouver) incorporated both aspects when he said, "I think prayer comes from a very deep, authentic, emotive, and rational place."

Prayer as Political

Sociologist and Asian studies scholar Anna Sun (2016, 122) describes prayer as "made possible only through the triangular relationship among the self, society, and the divine, with society as the mediating force." Acts of prayer are shaped by self and social ties that are in turn shaped by societal structures – social, religious, economic, and political – that are imbued with power. Prayer could externalize struggles that participants experienced in the everyday, such as financial hardship and immigration difficulties that were linked to the effects of government policies. The ritual of prayer could thus be perceived as an act of agency that could help participants deal with liminal states of prosperity and deprivation, belonging and marginalization. For example, a prayer request written into a prayer book in the chapel articulated these concerns: "Now please help me that Clara will be given her working visa to come here to take care of my grandchildren. Also, please help me financially abundantly. In Jesus' name, I pray and claim this now." Prayer could be "treated as part of one's religious *habitus*, a set of external rules and practices internalized by the individual through long processes of conscious and unconscious socialization" (Sun 2016, 125) and therefore a source of release and comfort in the face of difficult circumstances, giving spiritual sustenance and support.

However, prayer as part of one's religious *habitus* could be perceived and experienced as oppressive. Whether because of personal histories, adverse experiences with religion, or perceiving majoritarian religions as repressive and abusive, not all participants thought of prayer positively, but could view it as "coercive" and harmful (Woodhead 2015b, 220). While meanings ascribed to prayer were, for the most part, deeply personal and meaningful for the participants in our study, any understanding of the meaning and specialness of prayer should be held in balance with those situations in which it was absent or unwelcomed. Stella, an administrator in Vancouver, told us, "It might be my own stuff. If you ask every person 'Would you like to pray?,' it feels like 'No, don't push that on me.'" Participants who had grown up with negative experiences of religion, or those of Indigenous backgrounds could find such a context (where the majoritarian religion remained dominant) difficult in making known their preferences. Some participants of minority faith traditions and nones felt that their prayer traditions and forms of spirituality were not acknowledged because of uneven availability of representation in the healthcare settings, even though an organization could honour a multi-faith ethos, where everyone is valued (Reimer-Kirkham and Cochrane 2016; Sharma and Reimer-Kirkham 2015).

ON EXPRESSING PRAYER

Now we turn to how prayer was expressed, transitioning from conceptual meanings to specific ways of enacting prayer. We consider four overlapping areas (form, substance, process, and function), answering several questions: What form did prayer take? What did people include in their prayer? How did prayer come about? What does prayer do? In each area, we have attempted to show a range of social relations at play, such that both inclusive and exclusive dynamics are made evident.

Form

What form did prayer take? Form is usually defined as the configuration of something or a particular way in which a thing exists. The multiple forms of prayer in our study mapped loosely onto the dimensions of (1) formal and informal, (2) collective and individual, and (3) religious and non-religious. These dimensions turned out not to be bounded, but rather operated as loose classifications, with people moving in and out and between them. The variations within these dimensions were remarkable, showing prayer as personal, contextual, and intentional. Indeed, we were struck by the multiple forms prayer took, even as religion's influence in both Canada and England continues to decline.

We understood formal prayer as corporate or liturgical prayers, and informal prayer as unscripted prayers. Formal prayers were part of services (such as Catholic Mass) and special celebrations, such as Ash Wednesday. They were typically set prayers, like Muslim *Salat*, the Lord's Prayer or *Keshal* chanting, and might well involve some protocol (as in an Indigenous healing ceremony). As one would expect in a hospital, hospice, or care home, they also included the Christian sacrament of Anointing of the Sick. Matteo, a priest in Vancouver, showed us the small case in which he carried the elements, as he made his rounds to offer Holy Communion to bed-bound patients (see chapter 8). For many, formal prayers from their religious traditions were deeply significant.

In contrast, informal prayers were unstructured and spontaneous. For example, "If you are in peace and truthful to yourself and to the spirit, that is prayer" (Aurelia, citizen, London). Some prayers were uniquely crafted as a "way to lift up the current situation" (Ronald, chaplain, Vancouver). Listening was an important part of informal prayers, to the extent that prayer could be "listening to someone's story" (Chen, healthcare professional, Vancouver). Sometimes informal prayers took uncommon forms, as in the description by one chaplain of the "prayer puffs" (Jane, chaplain, Vancouver) she employed as a means of "sending a little prayer your way," such as to anxious waiting family members. Informal prayers were also expressed in the case of dance and music coming together in the enactment of prayer, for example, while listening to Andrea Bocelli's song "Prayer."

Collective and individual prayers were also described. They were said at the beginning of a board meeting in Vancouver, or the Christian fellowship held weekly in the London chapel. Collective prayers happened in the viewing room near the morgue, when Andreas chanted in the presence of family and their deceased loved one to release the expression of grief and emotions. Individual prayers were those of a chaplain said silently entering the hospital at the start of the day, or a Muslim doctor slipping into the multi-faith space in London to say prayers. Some of these individual prayers were non-verbal; as Frances, a chaplain in Vancouver put it, "Prayer is breathing."

Prayer could be religious and non-religious. Religious prayers were understood as located within a religious tradition, whether Buddhist, Catholic, or Sikh, and so on. Non-religious prayers were less likely to be restricted by religious forms and instead were directed to "the beyond," "the universe," or more immanently embedded in day-to-day routines, viewing art or being in nature. Prayer can be viewed as in-between, especially by those who identify as non-religious (Drescher 2016). Such "praying between the lines" could encompass many things, forms, relationships, and histories, blurring religious and non-religious traditions and rituals. The chapter's opening narrative reflects an in-betweenness relating to formal and informal prayer (something Anna-lise describes as a "ritual" but that has an impromptu feel rather than a set form), and to the group who gathered (with a "Roman Catholic, a Christian, a Hindu, someone 'spiritual but not religious,' our Buddhist Registered Nurse and me").

Substance

Next, we consider the substance of prayer. What did people include in their prayers? One way to study this is in the prayer request books found in churches, cathedrals, shrines, and hospitals. Several scholars have investigated prayer request books. Sociologists Wendy Cadge and M. Daglian examined "what kinds of requests people make of God and how they construct God in their prayers" (2008, 358). Religious studies scholar Tania ap Siôn (2015) analyzed prayer requests in an English cathedral to establish a framework for intercessory prayer. Social anthropologist Peter Collins gathered 3,000 prayer requests from hospitals in the northeast of England to conceptualize how they might "shed light on 'religion' and 'spirituality' in the UK in the twenty-first century" (2015, 192). In our research, prayer request books and cards placed in the formally designed hospital-designated sacred spaces were typically well-used. They were a place for people to write down their good news, but also their cares, apprehensions, anxieties, and uncertainties. Consider these examples: "Thank you. Please look after my son. Please help all my kids," and "Jesus, bless my family with health. Bless my sons with good marks in their education. Praise you Lord."

In addition to prayer requests, for those performing prayer on behalf of others, the substance of prayer meant expressing vulnerability in another way, where they revealed themselves and the sincerity of their beliefs and hopes for patients and their loved ones. Taryn (chaplain, Vancouver) explained: "What's so touching about prayer for me is it's this space where I don't need to pretend anymore. With a patient it's a place where we can express honestly our hope for them, for their families, for their well-being." Sometimes chaplains felt uncomfortable when asked to pray for healing or a cure, especially in the face of what seemed to be medical futility. In these cases, they balanced praying as requested with not feeding into unrealistic hope. As one chaplain said, "It's prayer of demand. We ask for things for ourselves and for others." Prayer, then, was being with a patient who was physically weak and exposed and the chaplain mirroring that through self-revealing in the substance of the prayer. The meaning of prayer was considered an honest act of disclosing oneself and sharing one's hopeful intentions for another. Within these examples of the substance of prayer, where meaningfulness was found in reaching out to connect to a higher being or to another person, a sociology of prayer takes place. Through the content of prayers there is an entering into or being in relationship with the other, the heart of prayer itself (Stringer 2015).

Process

The social relations of prayer were entwined with the process of prayer, such as why it emerged in the first place (motivations) and how prayer came about, including the conditions in which prayer was offered. Sociologist Michael Mason (2013) observes that the most common motive for prayer cited by theorists and researchers is that of seeking worldly benefits, whether protection from harm or for health, wealth, and success. These motives were evident in our project (portrayed in the foregoing Substance section), but we were as interested in non-material, non-petitionary processes of prayer that revolved around motivations of duty (related to religious identity) and seeking spiritual goals (for example, self-effacement through contemplation). The notion of process drew our attention to four influences on how prayer came about: religious identity; presenting circumstances; concerns for person-centredness and permission; and privacy.

First, the process of prayer highlighted the norms and expectations of religious identity that still exist as motivation for prayer (see chapter 7). Chaplains and staff alike referenced their religious identity as reason to pray, with comments such as, "I'm a practising Catholic, so prayer is my way of communicating, of expressing my commitment to my faith." Similarly, Chen commented, "My managers know that I'm a Muslim. I have to pray, I have to fast." Ezra told us, "In the Jewish faith, you have different prayers for different occasions. There are the daily prayers, there are the prayers for the Sabbath, the prayers for the holidays, and then there's also prayers for people who are sick. There are different kind of prayers, different psalms, different prayers. Why do I pray? Because I think that it's important, because I connect to God, because of tradition, because I love my faith" (chaplain, London). Sociologist Robert Wuthnow argues that prayer is "a learned behaviour ... typically embedded in the practices of religious traditions.... [F]rom earliest times prayers have been reported, preserved, and passed from generation to generation" (2008, 334–5). Like the above participants explained, the process and practice of prayer is linked to religious tradition and identity. Prayer could therefore be felt as both reward and obligation: "Prayer. Sometimes it's a real effort [*laughs*]. You don't feel like it, you just think, 'Oh gosh, I should pray.' But if you do pray, usually something happens and it becomes less difficult.... I was brought up a Roman Catholic and there's a bit in me of 'You must say your prayers.' It's a slightly different emphasis for me, now being Anglican. But there's a bit of that in me. You know, 'I must jabble my prayers every morning [*laughs*], otherwise God is going to be angry with me'" (Kirstie, citizen, London).

Second, the context of healthcare appeared to shift motivations for prayer. As important as religious identity and tradition were as reasons to pray, chaplains told us that the most common reason to request prayers related to crisis and death, when all types of existential concerns were wrapped up into expressions of prayer. Zara, a London healthcare professional, explained her observations of the reasons for prayer among patients: "When people become ill, their religious and spiritual needs become heightened because that's when they're searching for answers, solutions, and looking for hope. When you're living in fear, that's when you're turning to God and your faith to find the answers to your problems." Annalise's opening scenario of the room-blessing illustrates prayer as specific to the circumstances one finds oneself in and reflects an existential concern that "the spirits need permission and assistance to leave" after death.

Third, the social nature of prayer was a strong theme, especially with the condition that prayer be patient-led or person-centred. Chaplains took their cue from patients and families when performing prayer, according to one reflection: "You take your cues from the situation, the environment, the people within that space. There's an element of permission to pray. You ask, 'What does prayer mean to you?' I'm in spaces where people don't know what they want, what to do. They're caught, they're numb, they're in shock. And yet I'm not afraid to ask the question whether prayer is an option" (Taryn, chaplain). From this excerpt, we observed that the process of prayer comes about by seeking permission and determining whether the patient wanted prayer. However, person-centredness was sometimes overlooked. Curtis shared his perspectives on facilitating prayer:

When somebody says, "Can you bring me a bowl of water, so I can pray?," in response someone asks, "Why do you need a bowl of water to pray?" If you were a Muslim person, you need that to ritually purify yourself before going in to prayer. It is a necessary thing. And that request takes on a whole different meaning. There's so much around power and authority and prejudice or perceptions of prejudice. Many people who are newcomers to

Canada are not very comfortable asserting their needs. They're not as likely to be as direct in their requests. And we're a society that says, "If you want it, you have to ask for it. If you don't ask, you don't get."

In this case, the intersecting relations of power at individual, institutional, and societal levels prevented prayer from happening. By far the majority of descriptions in our data were those of prayer offered in careful, person-centred ways to patients and families, but a close reading of the data revealed times when patients and families could be left to their own devices for prayer or simply ignored, or conversely, openness to prayer could be assumed, apart from a person-centred philosophy (as was the case where a healthcare professional offered prayer to all her patients).

There was variation amongst healthcare professionals in their understanding of whether professional standards and codes of ethics allowed prayer with patients. Social workers, therapists, and physicians were less concerned with professional boundaries to prayer, with one physician going as far as "prescribing prayer." In both Vancouver and London, nurses as compared to other healthcare professionals, were less likely to expect that they would engage in prayer with a patient. Their ambivalences might well have to do with variation in what they were taught about spirituality, spiritual care-giving, and prayer. Undoubtedly the public cases in Britain[1] of nurses being disciplined on account of praying with patients also influenced how permission was perceived. While these cases demonstrate the sensitivity around prayer in healthcare settings, the NHS (Donnelly 2017) is suggesting that nurses and doctors must not be afraid to ask patients about their spiritual, cultural, religious, and social preferences.

Fourth, with permission in place, privacy became another important condition for prayer. Clinical settings such as hospitals are notorious for their lack of privacy, and chaplains, staff, and patients needed to find ways to work around this. We had a conversation with Matteo, a priest, about prayer happening at the bedside:

MATTEO: When there are two, three, four patients, they feel a little uncomfortable.
RESEARCHER: Yes. So what do you do?
MATTEO: Close the door, the curtains around the bed. And sometimes the patient asks to go to a private room. But if the patient

likes being in their bed better, then I tell them to speak slowly,
and I quietly [pray]. They quietly say what they want [prayer
for].... But I know that when you pray for a person, others listen.... It's also good then because people will feel with the others
and feel involved in prayer, in harmony. But there is no privacy as
such, especially with four patients in a room.

Closed doors and curtains helped to create separate and personal
spaces, but others were often within close proximity. Prayers at the
bedside meant that some patients and chaplains talked quietly to one
another, leaning in or over to hear and communicate. Niall (chaplain,
Vancouver) put it this way: "Recognizing the sacredness of prayer, I
wouldn't want to pray in a patient eating lounge where there is talking and noise, as that does not seem very sacred. I always try to have
some privacy, quiet, and confidentiality." With this desire for privacy, it
was fascinating that prayer often occurred in very public ways and
places – in corridors, in elevators, and in waiting rooms. As Matteo
explained, not all prayer is private. What seemingly is a private
moment becomes public with others listening in. Thus the social relations of prayer are not only between a person and higher being or
between two people, but a collective occurrence in which others
could participate. Prayer then transgressed the constraints placed
between private and public and in a seemingly secular medical context (see chapters 2 and 9).

Function

I was talking to the guy in the gift shop, and there was another guy in the
gift shop, who is doing our gift shop construction, who has a brand-new
daughter, who is not doing very well and had surgery last Friday. I said to
him, "I can get the nuns to pray for her." And he looked at me a little star-
tled. I said, "Hey, you never know." And he looked at me and he said, "That
would be great, thanks." And I said, "What's her name?" And he said her
name. So the sisters prayed for her last Friday, and you know what, I think it
made him feel much better. I think the sisters have more pull.

Sharon, administrator, Vancouver

Related to the form, substance, and process of prayer is the function
of prayer, what it does. In the foregoing excerpt, prayer was offered
because of what it was perceived to do, to provide healing for his

daughter and comfort to the father during a time of uncertainty. The function of prayer relates to instrumentality; Mason explains that when prayer is defined as instrumental, "prayer is not an end in itself but a means to other ends" (2013, 12).

Prayer could function in several ways. First, story was an important element of prayer, providing a way for people to disclose their circumstances to another. Liam, a healthcare professional in Vancouver, shared that "a First Nations woman, around Christmas time, a really hard time for her, was telling me her story, and it was almost like a confession or prayer, she was remembering and reminiscing about her father."

Second, the act of telling one's story, being heard in the presence of another can also be a deep comfort. A former patient told us, "I found comfort at my worst time through prayer" (Lata, London). Prayer's function was a way to experience consolation during grief. Ersi, a healthcare professional in London, explained the long history of prayer in her life and how it functioned as a source of comfort: "From childhood, I have learned [prayers] in Arabic. Now I have the Quran translated in English. I have never thought about translating it or it wouldn't have stayed in my head. There is something comforting about repeating, it's almost like a mantra. You know the words, they've been with you all your life, you just repeat. And so prayer is about returning to a comforting place." The repetitive function of prayer, to say words over and over again, that one has learned from a young age, provided comfort and connection to personal, familial, and religious histories that travel with people from place to place and over time.

Third, prayer provided a way to seek guidance: "It's to give guidance through your day, provide direction on how you want to live your life ... clarity. That's how I find prayer to be" (Keith, healthcare professional, Vancouver). This kind of prayer could "allow reality and different interpretations of reality" (Woodhead 2015b, 225). The practice of prayer challenged a single subjectivity by making room for a God, spirit, higher being, or another to enter in and "to speak as one's inner voice" (225). Prayer's function to guide could result in "changing the subject" (Woodhead 2015b), allowing one to view circumstances differently.

Fourth, prayer also bonded and brought families, patients, and staff together. It could build bridges, connect across difference, and function as social capital (Bramadat 2005; Putnam 2000). Family prayed for their loved ones: "The son who was visiting seeing his father was from the UK and a health professional. Yesterday there were both the son and the chaplain together united in prayer" (Frances, chaplain, Vancouver). Family members from beyond the grave were also said to take part. A family said that their deceased grandmother had requested prayer. Patients prayed for staff. Jane described a shared moment of prayer: "At one point, she (patient) raised her hand in the air, her palm facing outward, and I thought perhaps this was to 'high five' me. I automatically lifted my hand up to meet hers and she took it, wrapped her fingers around mine and in the most natural of movements, we joined our other hand together and she broke into leading open prayer with me." Patients also prayed for other patients. "When I visited, she was never alone. While she was able, she was very happy to pray with me, and the offer was extended to whoever else was there" (Paul, chaplain, London). And staff prayed for each other. In one situation, healthcare professionals and the chaplain described "huddling together" like a sports team before a game to say prayers for a particularly stressful situation faced by a family. Some staff sought out quiet time for prayer in chapel spaces. Surgeons often used the chapel before surgery to pray or reflect. Other healthcare professionals offered silent prayers for patients who were suffering; in the words of a participant, "I pray on my own for a patient, and when I'm with patients, silently in my mind I will pray, and I'll do that on my own if someone's really struggling and I don't know how to help them" (Ameena, Vancouver). Who prays, and for whom, sheds light on both familiar and unexpected occurrences of prayer between people.

Fifth, prayer can also be misplaced or have harmful effect. For all of the stories in this book that speak to the connecting power of prayer, prayer needed to be heeded in a way that did not silence or shut down a meaningful exchange. Alexia told us, "A lot of our residents or staff members, all they want to do is talk. They don't necessarily want to hear a prayer. They want to talk to you about something. Or they want to be heard. And that's very different from a prayer. When you have a resident who's just moved in, who's in a very sensitive state, crying, I don't think that she or he wants to hear a prayer. I think he or she just wants to be heard" (administrator, Vancouver). She described how listening was important to residents and those newly transitioning into long-term care. Prayer could therefore be misplaced or misjudged as needed, even though it might be done out of care by a staff member. Other healthcare staff and chaplains expressed angst about offering prayer, afraid of it being misperceived or causing unintended harm. An excerpt from Martin's research diary captures this sentiment:

> Attending a place of worship is the right and the choice of a patient in that environment. The patient (who had severe mental health issues) had chosen to attend a Christmas Day service. I prayed for caution for myself. Anything I did or said could have had a negative consequence to that man's life. I could have been at fault for saying the wrong thing, or by holding a wrong intent present in the circumstances, even if unarticulated. I could have been misinterpreted with a negative connotation. As I offered prayer, I have never been more afraid of a catastrophic consequence.

Martin was highly tuned to the fact that the words used for prayer could cause distress or personal harm, especially to someone with a mental illness. Similarly, Ersi talked about how prayer could conjure unwanted feelings that have caused much suffering, or prayer could be perceived as forcing one's values on another: "Prayers can be damaging for people when they come from a critical parental voice which reinforces shame or feeling bad about yourself, guilt, all of those things." Other people, even those who were devout, might simply not be interested in prayer. In the words of John (administrator, London), "Prayer is part of spiritual care, but only where it is appropriate."

TRANSGRESSION AND PRAYER

What do these meanings and expressions of prayer in healthcare settings tell us about religion in the public sphere? Prayer transgressed categories such as public/private and religious/non-religious. Prayer could also bridge individuals and collectives, and it could transgress difference by connecting and distancing. The social relations of prayer described by participants could be both inclusive and exclusive. Yet the expansive nature of the social relations of prayer meant that it could counter societal messages that emphasize that individuals alone are responsible for their circumstances. In reality, everyday lives intersect, and the social act of prayer brought to light hurtful and hopeful realities. Prayer was not neutral. It was personal and also political, externalizing and mediating the wider social structures that participants were affected by.

While we present myriad prayer stories in this book, we caution against over-reading the presence of prayer and religion. For example, when we asked chaplains about how often they had prayed with patients in the past five days, their responses ranged from approximately once per day, to many times per day. Who the chaplain was, who the patients were, the particular circumstances facing them, and the broader context all shaped occurrences of prayer. Likewise, many other non-medical activities intended for healing, such as the wide array of complementary and alternative medicines, are engaged with in hospitals, but are not deemed as prayer. Many of these activities also transgress the rules of biomedicine and its associated clinical practices. Our analytic challenge, and the work of the chapters that follow, is to tease out what is unique and transgressive about prayer.

Creating an Inclusive Public Sphere: Healthcare and the Role of Prayer

Sheryl Reimer-Kirkham and Lori G. Beaman

It is often the case that in one room, there are four beds, four residents, four religions, and four languages.

Tulio, chaplain, Vancouver

My colleagues were dismissive, saying, "We don't pay you to pray."

Emina, healthcare professional, Vancouver

In this chapter we explore the co-constitution of prayer and the public sphere: what prayer in healthcare can reveal about religion in the public sphere, and how the public sphere of healthcare shapes spiritual practices such as prayer. A peculiar mix of state presence and personal intimacy, hospitals are multi-faceted social systems and microcosms of broader society where cooperation, ambivalence, and conflict coincide. The first quote above from one of the chaplains who participated in our study sets the scene and reveals much about the intimate spaces of healthcare, where the fragility of life intersects with a range of values, beliefs, and backgrounds. The second quote reveals divergent views on whether prayer belongs in the public sphere of healthcare, in a scenario where a nurse is scolded by her colleagues for praying with a patient. We witnessed intimacy and cooperation as well as conflict and disagreement in the context of diversity over and over again in our fieldwork in Canadian and English hospitals.

The varied and contested expressions of religious diversity in the public sphere of healthcare, including the naming of secular and sacred, are socially constructed realties of power relations, organized by broader social and historical forces. Our exploration of diversity in this chapter (and this book) draws from feminist critiques of diversity discourses that infer "benign variation … which bypasses power as well as history to suggest a harmonious empty pluralism" (Ahmed 2012, 13). We aim to think through those points at which relations of power meet, including a hospital or even a hospitalized person, for, as feminist scholar Sara Ahmed goes on to say, "A body can be a meeting point" (14). This project on religion in the public sphere, with its entrée of prayer, has turned out to be a remarkable location from which to examine such meeting points, from our vantage at three edges of the study of religion. First, the locations of Vancouver and London have meant our data collection occurred in two super-diverse, global cities, characterized by migration, emergent spiritualities, and non-religion, all forcing changes on dominant or majoritarian religions. As described in the Introduction, statistics for Vancouver report about 17 per cent affiliating with religions other than Christianity (compared to Canada's 9 per cent), and 41.5 per cent as nones (compared to Canada's 24 per cent; Statistics Canada 2011). A further salient influence in Vancouver is the imperative of reconciliation with Indigenous peoples who make up 4.9 per cent of Canada's population (Statistics Canada 2017a). London's "microclimate" (Bullivant 2017) is distinct from the religious affiliation of the rest of England; it is the most religious area of England, mainly because of its large Muslim and migrant communities, while also having a lower proportion of nones (31 per cent) than the rest of the country (48 per cent).

As a second edge of the study of religion, chaplaincy (the primary sample for our project) has been described as at the forefront of adapting to this changing face of religion (Bender 2014; Woodhead 2015a). Chaplains often have to formulate answers to questions the institutional churches have not yet begun to ask (Gilliat-Ray 1999, as quoted in Eccles 2014, 9; Woodhead 2015a). Their work has been described as liminal (see chapter 5) both in relation to their place on multidisciplinary healthcare teams, and their work at the margins of the church and the secular institutions by whom they are employed (Eccles 2014; Norwood 2006; Threlfall-Holmes and Newitt 2011a). This marginal position may create an opportunity to transgress another space "between the orthodox and that secular space that was previously considered taboo" (Eccles 2014, 9). Anthropologist Courtney Bender (2014, n.p.) puts it this way: "Chaplains are on the cutting edge of elaborating a quasi-secular, medical and multi-faith use for prayers in modern medicine."

The third compelling edge is that of healthcare. This arena has not undergone the same critical scrutiny in regard to religious diversity compared to other public institutions (such as education or law). Because of their training, healthcare professionals are anchored in natural and clinical sciences, more so than arts and the humanities; corresponding assumptions about rationality, generalizability, and objectivity have left little acknowledgment of the sacred in clinical settings. Yet we wonder if there is perhaps something unique about healthcare in relation to the secular because of its proximity to suffering, illness, and death; whether it is safe from some of the negative effects of institutionalized (organized) religions; and whether we might derive new insights about deep equality here. Perhaps prompted by the immediacy and array of diversity (as reflected in the introductory quotation) in conjunction with the vulnerabilities of illness and suffering, we see in these hospital settings the beginnings of a more inclusive response to diversity.

Maintaining a critical interpretive lens has proved a constant challenge. We have reflected extensively on the character of the hospitals in our study in relation to the sacred and the secular, the private and the public. The hospitals have retained some of their religious or sacred character in their transition from being privately supported institutions to publicly funded components of the state apparatus (explained in more detail below) that is often blurred, with prayer having the capacity to transgress assumptions about the secular. We have also been well aware of the draw of a "will to religion" (Beaman 2013) throughout this project, most specifically the idea that we all have spiritual needs. We have questioned the extent to which the will to religion is represented by a confessional, panoptic spirituality that invites assessment of the patient's spiritual needs (see Sullivan 2014), and any expectation that prayer would be welcome for most. At the same time, we recognize the genuine caring and responsiveness of those who offer spiritual care in the healthcare setting. We are on tricky ground, indeed, exploring a wide-ranging spectrum of needs and desires with prayer at the centre.

To tend to the politics of difference at play in the public sphere of healthcare, we have benefitted from sociologist James Beckford's (2014) mapping of the analytic dimensions of diversity: we describe empirical forms of diversity in relation to religion in the first section on theorizing diversity; we trace normative positions about the value of diversity in section two on historicizing diversity in healthcare; we present legal/social policies regulating religion in a section on managing religious diversity; and finally we home in on the relational contexts of everyday interactions, what we refer to as "living diversity," to show how new diversity is worked out at the point of care. Drawing on the notion of deep equality (Beaman 2017a, 2017b), we explore notions of agonistic respect, caring, and generosity to trace the ways that social actors work through difference in the highly charged atmospheres of hospitals.

THEORIZING THE PUBLIC SPHERE

The public sphere is generally conceptualized as what belongs to the state, the domain that is regulated by legislation and policy and typically comprises institutions that are state-funded (e.g., healthcare, education, law). In the case of our research sites, by merit of their state funding with government oversight and public accountabilities, they clearly fall into this category of "public sphere." Interestingly, the relevance of the concept of public sphere to the day-to-day functioning of these hospitals goes largely unexamined, unless religion is involved. Then, current discourses on public spaces as secular are invoked, with attending questions about the nature of the public sphere, the meaning of the secular, and boundaries between public and private. These discourses were evident as shaping the social relations of prayer as we came to understand them within this project. Some participants in our study fully supported a widespread uptake of prayer in healthcare settings; others had the opposite perspective, with a view that prayer (and other spiritual practices) had little place in the public sphere of healthcare. For example, a hospital in England declined participation because our study was deemed "too religious" for a "secular" hospital, inferring a publicly funded National Health Service (NHS) hospital as a neutral place devoid of religious expression. Another participant mused that it was surprising that spiritual care services were even allowed in a NHS hospital. These examples surface the enigma of how religion (and prayer) in the public sphere is understood, and, as introduction to this terrain, in this section we offer a short primer on the public sphere and secularism. While this will be familiar ground for many, such discussion remains largely absent from healthcare literatures on religious diversity.

The work of philosopher and sociologist Jürgen Habermas is a common starting point for understanding the public sphere. In brief, a Habermasian ([1962] 1989) conception of the public sphere, built on the social change of the Renaissance, invites an understanding of the public sphere as more than a conflation with state apparatuses or economic markets. He coined the term *public sphere* to designate a theatre in modern societies in which political participation is enacted through talk. Despite this early signal to democratic, civic spaces of engagement, what has evolved in large part, including in Canadian and English contexts, is the construction of the public sphere as a constitutional, legislative, and political arena. With such a reading, boundaries between public and private are construed as relatively impermeable, and solutions to conflicts or perceived incompatibilities tend to be procedural or legislative, with law framing responses to diversity in terms of reasonable accommodation. This framing has migrated into the public sphere, permeating everyday responses to religious diversity. Consider this comment from Elizabeth, a London chaplain who identified as a person of faith, but was careful to not bring that aspect of herself to her practice: "I work with a Muslim lady, and she goes and has her prayer time, and we accommodate all of that, which is only right. Her faith is overt and the organization adapts to that, but they don't make any adaption to me as a Christian. But then I don't ask for it I suppose." In this invocation of accommodation, the "Muslim lady" is constructed as an Other to be accommodated and the diversity she presents as something to be managed (Beaman 2012; Reimer-Kirkham and Cochrane 2016). Moreover, although Elizabeth says that it is "only right" that her Muslim co-worker be accommodated, she positions herself as somehow being excluded from "adaptation" as a Christian. Elizabeth is not clear what would be required for such an adaptation, nor does she recognize her relative position of privilege or the inherent hierarchy constructed by the accommodation framework (Selby, Barras, and Beaman 2018).

Notions of the secular are deployed in relation to the public sphere in varied ways. Modernity has brought a rhetoric of "the secular" in relation to a public sphere that is devoid of religion, and public institutions that are no longer in need of or interested in maintaining a "sacred cosmos or maintaining a public religious worldview" (Taylor 2007, 37). There has been a concomitant and varied engagement with the secular[1] as alternatively an achieved fact, a goal to be reached or an exclusionary force that prevents the full participation of all. Put otherwise, there are those who mobilize the secular nature of health-care as a social fact that governs and should govern how services are offered, and there are those who deploy it to decry the exclusive nature of social institutions such that religion is marginalized. Yet, while the secular and secularization are often frameworks within which hospitals and healthcare are understood, this framing obscures the social processes and relations that occur. We thus bracket the sec-ular as a fact, a goal or exclusionary force and instead focus on the everyday interactions of social actors in the healthcare system. While not ignoring their invocations of the secular, we have not assumed the secular a priori, but rather have considered it through the experiences of individuals and collectives. Ronald, a Vancouver chaplain, mused about the secular in healthcare settings: "We are secular. We are spiri-tual at the same time. I don't see a wall between the secular and the sacred. The last thing I want is to create another silo."

Local actors thus may be more flexible, engaged, and creative. They may achieve a positive resolution of conflict or disagreement in inno-vative ways. While formal regulations often depend on a rigid con-ceptualization of identities (whether around religion, ethnicity, gen-der, or sexuality), informal processes are less likely to reify identity and are better able to respond to the intersectional way in which identity is lived. We suggest that the conceptualization of deep equality (Bea-man 2017a, 2017b) can be a mode by which to create an accessible public sphere. Deep equality is characterized by respect, neighbourli-ness, and caring, values and actions enacted in informal ways by indi-vidual actors in the public sphere (see chapter 7), as well as embedded in institutions' (such as healthcare) missions, values, and policies (dis-cussed in chapter 4). Through the lens of deep equality, social rela-tions in the public sphere are seen not primarily as legislative or legal matters but rather as matters of ethics and relationality – an approach well suited to the public sphere of healthcare.

In our study, far from being public spaces stripped of religious expression, a range of religious and non-religious expression was pre-sent in the everyday and needed to be worked out. A chaplain new to the role put it this way: "In terms of religious diversity ... I've only been here four months, so just take that into consideration.... I've encountered people of Buddhist faith, a few of Jewish faith, certainly Christian faith. I have provided support to people of First Nations spirituality. But probably the biggest category are people who will assert that they are spiritual but not religious" (Niall, chaplain, Vancouver). This level of diversity meant that a wide range of spiritual and religious needs were evident in the settings we studied: after death, the body of a Buddhist patient is requested to be left in the hospital room for twelve to twenty-four hours so that the spirit could have a peaceful exit; washing facilities (basin of water) are provided for a bed-bound Sikh patient prior to his prayers; a healing ceremony with Indigenous smudging in the designated, ventilated First Nations sacred space; Muslim prayers with a mat facing Mecca and staff fasting during Ramadan; a South Asian matriarch with fifty visitors, with a community faith leader supporting prayers; a Wiccan patient seeking spiritual support; a Catholic priest visiting a bedside to offer the sacrament of the sick; an Orthodox chaplain chanting to ritualize death. Unquestionably the public space of these hospitals included citizens and staff who brought with them their religious and non-religious practices.

Even as civic spaces, however, it is unlikely that public spheres in general, and healthcare specifically, are ever fully accessible or welcoming to everyone. Exchange may be uneven, imbued with power relations and imbalances that are not readily discernible. Public spaces are sites of enforcement, resistance, cooperation, collaboration, exclusion, and inclusion. Though formal regulations such as laws can provide greater access to the public sphere and protect actors within it, and indeed can shift the very boundary of what is designated as public, equally important are navigations and negotiations undertaken by actors who create spaces of meaningful equality. Often power relations are structured by historical contingencies that lie just below the surface. It is to those that we now turn.

HISTORICIZING RELIGION AND HEALTHCARE

In order to better understand the shape of current articulations of diversity, we highlight a core development in each context we studied, illustrating the traces of the past intermarriage between religious and state powers. In Vancouver, as elsewhere across Canada, the history of colonial church-run residential schools has left a profoundly negative, intergenerational legacy on Indigenous peoples, as over a period of more than 100 years children were forcibly separated from their families to be indoctrinated into the culture of the legally dominant Euro-Christian Canadian society (TRC 2015). The Truth and Reconciliation Commission (begun in 2009 with the final report presented to the federal government in 2015), with its mandate to inform all Canadians about what happened in the Indian residential schools, has created a historical account and generated ninety-four calls to action, seven of which are targeted specifically to healthcare, to redress the legacy of residential schools and advance Canadian reconciliation. Many Indigenous people access healthcare services which serve as a daily "contact zone" reminiscent of the colonial powers wielded by church-run residential schools, and thus a patient's Indigenous identity might be positioned vis-à-vis the religious identity of a healthcare organization, as reflected by Shannon (healthcare professional, Vancouver): "Aboriginal people certainly don't appreciate the church because of residential trauma, school trauma, and things like that. I try to steer away from that and say, 'This is a place where we want to heal your heart as well as heal your body, and there are people here who can pray with you, that can listen to you.' I really try not to talk a lot about Christianity, especially in front of an Aboriginal person." When we asked an Indigenous elder who provided healing ceremonies for hospitalized Indigenous patients about what it meant for a religiously affiliated healthcare setting to be providing services to many Indigenous people, she provided a poignant, one-word answer: "Redemption." This word references the harms that were historically perpetrated by the church, while also signalling the current mandate of reconciliation. As with many other Canadian institutions, this particular site is making efforts to de-colonize its approaches to healthcare service delivery. The creation of a First Nations sacred space (described in chapter 3), a team devoted to Indigenous well-being, and a recent healing ceremony to mark a new partnership between Indigenous and religiously affiliated organizations are three examples. The challenge will be to integrate reconciliation and respect into all caregiving encounters with Indigenous patients, as a way of transcending the past.

In England the historical presence of the Church of England in the NHS also continues, albeit with a trajectory of decline. The state church, with continued representation of unelected bishops in Parliament, has been described as less in step with the public's views (e.g., on female episcopal ordination and same-sex marriage) as attendance has dwindled. Christian chaplaincy has served as a longstanding presence of the Church of England in the secular context of the NHS, with many appointed chaplains also ordained ministers (Pattison 2015; Swift 2015). A transition to multi-faith chaplaincy evolved after the

2000 Orchard Report that was critical of Christian chaplains acting as brokers for other religious traditions (see chapter 5). More recently the NHS published a national guideline (NHS 2015) obligating pastoral support and care to non-religious people. Humanists UK (formerly the British Humanist Association) has long advocated for this shift to more accurately represent the citizenry of England, and as indicated on their website, to ensure non-religious people have access to pastoral support that reflects their world view, provided by like-minded individuals. One of our London sites had secured the services of a humanist chaplain who described her role with patients as vital but who also perceived herself as marginalized on the chaplaincy team with a dominance of chaplains affiliated with organized religions, with a Church of England majority. The National Secular Society in England has been a vocal critic of the NHS's funding of chaplains, and this sentiment was also expressed in our study by Stanley, an administrator: "If you ask me about whether prayer is transgressive, yes. In a publicly funded system, chaplaincy is. But then you might say, 'Well with somebody with no religion, I regard this as essentially a private matter, and not to do with what the state should be doing one way or the other.' [The NHS] should have a permissive role. We should not have a facilitatory role in quite the way that we've adopted it. If I was a patient and I knew that there was a chaplain in on our inter-disciplinary team meeting, I'd be pretty cross." These examples of reconciliation with Canada's Indigenous populations and England's Humanist and Secularist critics underline the salience of understanding the provision of spiritual care services and the expression of prayer in hospital settings as taking place in an evolving public sphere that carries historic influences of majoritarian religions including close state-church relations, while simultaneously reflecting a range of contemporary expressions of religion and non-religion.

MANAGING DIVERSITY:
THE WORK OF HOSPITALS

Another angle or lens through which to examine religion in the public sphere in our case is that of how religious diversity is managed in hospital settings. Our research sites evidenced different ways of approaching diversity – specifically religious, generic, and inclusive approaches – that overlapped at the same site. Each approach contains traces of majoritarian religion, and each acknowledges the necessity of creating an inclusive atmosphere. The religious approach aligns with both pastoral care, where (virtually) all spiritual care is provided by the founding religious group to all patients (the exceptions might be specific religious rituals) and multi-faith chaplaincy, where a denomination or faith group provides spiritual care particular to their tradition. Public signage and website materials at one Vancouver site refer to pastoral care. Another study setting in Vancouver operated within a multi-faith model, with two paid chaplains (affiliated with Christian traditions) and a variety of volunteers representing Sikh, Hindu, Muslim, Indigenous, and Buddhist traditions. The multi-faith chaplaincy model at a London hospital illustrates the NHS move to create space for other religions beyond the Christian faith, such as including a Muslim chaplain and Humanist chaplain volunteer on the team. Bioethicist Trevor Stammers and theologian and sociologist Stephen Bullivant (2012) equate the multi-faith approach with the "common ground" model of secularism, explaining that this model "seeks to mediate between competing religious interests in the public square by opening up shared, ecumenical space to which all may contribute on an equal footing.... The key motivation here is that no one religion or denomination should be unduly privileged over any or all others" (86). The historical influence of founding religious groups, however, complicate the ideal of equal footing. Also contributing to the continued dominance of majoritarian (Christian) religion was the balance of religious affiliation of spiritual health practitioners and volunteers at both sites, with the majority self-identifying as Christian. Such dominance was also evident at some religiously affiliated sites with the presence of crosses and other religious iconography in hospital and meeting rooms (a point we return to below). Stammers and Bullivant (2012) assert that the real challenge in the common ground model is that in order to be inclusive, the inherited model – which is embedded in a society that was informed by a majoritarian Christian religious culture – must be replaced with something new.

A generic or universalist model of spiritual care has emerged as an alternative to the historic model of pastoral care and contemporary multi-faith chaplaincy, and this model too was present (alongside the multi-faith model) at some of our London and Vancouver sites. This generic approach is the preferred model put forward by the Canadian Association for Spiritual Care and British Columbia's Spiritual Health Advisory. The primary distinction from a multi-faith model is an emphasis not on religious traditions, but rather on a shared spirituality common to humanity. This approach has opened up spiritual care for all, regardless of whether they align with a faith tradition or not, as reflected by the earlier comment about the majority of spiritual care recipients being those who were "spiritual but not religious." However, critics of this approach have pointed to the problematic "will to religion" whereby spiritual needs are conferred on all, and others have voiced concern about the neutralizing effect that tends to erase specific identities (Beaman 2013; Coble 2018). As an example, in our study a hospitalized Indigenous youth would have valued having an Indigenous elder perform a healing ceremony but was not told this was available, although he was visited regularly by a (generic) spiritual health practitioner.

Our analysis of these approaches to managing diversity (i.e., the particularism of pastoral care and multi-faith chaplaincy, and the universalism of generic spirituality) at our study sites revealed, then, that each of these approaches could inadvertently exclude or silence groups of people. Our interest became examining the contours of the permissible, but also to then reflect more fully on the types of exclusion that might occur. During our discussions about what we were seeing in the data, we found ourselves engaged in a curious thought experiment: What if all spiritual care providers in hospitals were Wiccan? What if the chapel were reconfigured for inclusion with Wicca as a beginning place? We asked these questions not to be provocative, or to substitute one form of universalism with an imagined new form, but to attempt to shed light on the extent to which spiritual care is associated with Christianity, and how then prayer reflects the traces of Christianity that are laid bare by our thought experiment. In other words, what residual normative aspects of the Christian legacy remain in present-day expressions of what are often framed as generic spiritual care services? We were also interested in how these traces of Christianity infused the idea of the "public," particularly in relation to the folding in of the residue of Christianity with the ways in which the public is imagined. We were motivated by a concern for inclusivity, and struggling to sort through the intersection of "public" with a "religious" hospital (in the case of Canada), and remembering the historic influence of majoritarian religions (the Church of England and the Roman Catholic Church) on the NHS. We discussed the possibility that our framing of the project, through its emphasis on prayer, contained the universalizing tendencies identified by historian Daniel Boyarin and anthropologist Jonathan Boyarin (1993) in their reflec-

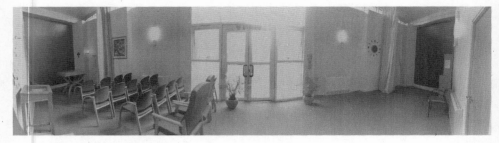

2.1　A multi-faith space

tions on the nature of Christianity: "The genius of Christianity is its concern for all the peoples of the world; the genius of Judaism is its ability to leave other people alone. And the evils of the two systems are the precise obverse of these genii. The genies all too easily become demons. Christian universalism, even at its most liberal and benevolent, has been a powerful force for coercive discourses of sameness, denying, as we have seen, the rights of Jews, women, and others to retain their difference" (707). Boyarin and Boyarin identify Judaism with particularism. We associate these two tendencies – sameness and *universalism*; difference and *particularism* – with some of the approaches to diversity we saw in our data. However, what most interested us was the emergence of something that we believe captures a third approach and is emerging in the new diversity. We see deep equality, and its emphasis on *similarity*, as a move between these two poles, that captures the complexities of who people are as they enter the healthcare setting. This tricky balancing of complexities is fraught with navigational hazards, which pull toward universalizing, "will to religion" (Beaman 2013) tendencies on the one hand and a drive to recognize difference that veers toward particularism on the other. Yet we observed an approach to diversity that is charting the course for the future that responds to a diverse landscape of multiple religious positions and none.

At one hospital, the designated sacred space had been configured to allow for a fluidity to accommodate Christians, Muslims, and the non-religious (see figure 2.1). At one end there is a simple Christian altar and a cross that can be hidden by curtains, and at the other end is a Muslim prayer area that can also be hidden by curtains. The rest of the space is free of any religious symbols, although there are windows overlooking a small garden and an art installation hung from the ceiling that could communicate spirituality-related concepts. Notably, a prayer board was located at the doorway to the sacred space (i.e., in the central, "neutral" zone), with multiple prayer requests pinned to it. Applying the concepts of deep equality, this space sidesteps imposition of universalism (sameness), allows for particularism (difference) where that might be necessary, and holds space for the non-religious. Perhaps most evocative about this configuration is the possibility of responsiveness to diversity, of fluidity in allowing an in-the-moment creation of inclusive space, simply by pulling curtains and re-arranging chairs. Indeed, this is what happens regularly, according to one participant who told us on one visit about conflict that had occurred earlier that day while Catholic Mass and Muslim prayers were occurring simultaneously: "The curtains are not really enough, but they always manage to work it out." In the last section of this chapter, we take up the analytic angle that has us looking closely to "lived diversity" in the context of prayer, allowing us to tease out those situations in which deep equality took form.

LIVING DIVERSITY: "WORKING IT OUT" AT THE POINT OF CARE

The main points of our argument thus far in this chapter are that the public sphere is a civic place of engagement, with historical residues and contemporary presences of institutionalized (majoritarian) religion at organizational levels; religion and non-religion enter into this public space through personal identities; organizational attempts to manage diversity in healthcare have traditionally been based on difference (particularism) or sameness (universalism); and there is some evidence of emerging models that account for new diversity and are thereby more inclusive. In this final section, we address two remaining questions: Can we elicit from a close look at how diversity is worked out in the everyday at the point of care a clearer sense of a truly inclusive (common ground) civic space? And, returning to our earlier question: Is there something unique about healthcare that shapes a different secularity that might inform us more broadly?

Reduced to its extremes, healthcare as a social institution and facet of the public sphere is shaped by life and death in ways that law or education, for example, are not. Also setting the healthcare domain apart from other social institutions and public spaces are the immediacy and unpredictability of access to the space, the intimacy and embodiment of the whole self in the engagement with the space, and the shared vulnerability encountered in facing the reasons that bring one into the space of requiring healthcare services (illness, social need, death). In London, Hannah, a former patient put it this way: "A hospital isn't a chosen private space.... [W]e don't get to choose when we have times of need." The experiences of illness and hospitalization often bring to the surface existential or sacred dimensions of life, in relation to deeper meanings, suffering, death, and afterlife. As a public sphere, then, healthcare is more apt to see the negotiation of religious/spiritual pluralism come to the fore, and we are more likely to encounter difference in ways that can be deeply meaningful and personal to people (e.g., what they hold close). Prayer in these times of crisis may be amplified or more common. Our claim is not that prayer is the pinnacle of spiritual connection or response to vulnerability; rather it emerged as one of a range of relational practices that was employed in navigating the complexities of diversity in times of illness, suffering, and vulnerability. In some situations, an offer of prayer or attendance at a prayer service (such as Friday Prayer for Muslims) provided comfort and connection. The multiplicity of prayer, when it occurred, gives insight into how the new diversity is worked out.

Intimacy and vulnerability are counterintuitive when we think about the public sphere, and yet they are both fundamentally linked to healthcare and to prayer. The notion of vulnerability is seldom associated with the public sphere, and it is worth thinking about more fully as something we can learn from those who work in healthcare.

> As for the vulnerability of patients, many have serious conditions, some have terminal illnesses. It doesn't really matter what background they come from, what faith or none, rich or poor, highly responsible jobs or homeless. They are all united in the fact that they need help and are dependent on a team of professionals to provide that help. Suddenly they find themselves out of their comfort zone, their dignity and self-control taken from them. Often in times of sickness or when facing death, people start to question life, its meaning and its purpose, and being in hospital gives people time to reflect. Respect and relationship with all our patients, irrespective of faiths or none, is what our ministry is about, and meeting people where they are gives back some dignity and control to the most vulnerable. (Wendy, chaplain, London)

We were repeatedly told that prayer had to occur within a framework of person-centredness, following the lead of the patient or person requesting prayer with a question such as, "How would you like me to pray?" As the most intimate of relational practices, prayer was approached by most of our participants with extreme caution. To be sure, we saw traces of universalism on occasion, but a comment from Taryn (chaplain, Vancouver) was more common:

I'm naturally very respectful to other people's traditions but not just faith traditions. Beliefs in general. Because I don't want to feel forced myself. I'm very cautious to engage in a way that if the table was turned and I was on the other side, and I was the vulnerable one because all of our clientele are in a vulnerable state, am I abusing that? That I have the privilege to go into their room, am I taking advantage of my power position with someone who is in a very weak space in their life right now? Or am I genuinely respecting them? And I think that would be the call of most healthcare or institutional organizations that would hire a spiritual health practitioner [chaplain], that we are willing to offer unconditional, positive regard and unconditional acceptance and be there to reflect that back to them, regardless of what they believe or whether they ask for prayer or reject it.

Taryn identifies a key element of the third way – that of seeking similarity – we identified in the foregoing section; rather than projecting spiritual need, the self-reflexive approach expressed here adopts a position of humility through the recognition of vulnerability. She went on to illustrate how this posture directed her to repeatedly visit a patient on the mental health unit, even though she sometimes dreaded the visit. "Her pain was up, she was an addict who was dirty and had expectations that I couldn't meet, that the staff couldn't meet. I found myself internally wanting to avoid her, but because of the referrals, I couldn't." After building a relationship of trust over many weeks (it turned out that they had the same birthday), one day the patient's first words were, "Will you pray with me?" The chaplain asked about how she might pray, and the patient said she "wanted to continue to experience God because he was showing up for her in the hospital." Shared prayer seemed to foster deeper trust, such that the patient "immediately just poured out her history, unprovoked." After several days of similar requests for prayer from the patient, the patient asked what her day looked like with "I'd like to pray for you too." "She grabbed my hand and she's praying and thanking God for me and her health and having the opportunity for us to get to know one another. Then, in the middle of the prayer, she stopped and said, 'God, thank you for her great nails' [*laughs*]." Taryn concluded, "I was just so moved by the authenticity of the whole experience and humbled by it. Her heart is purer than mine because it doesn't have this religiosity. She is just in that space, completely aware of her addictions, her weaknesses, her irritability ... with this very heartfelt, meaningful, non-traditional, affectionate prayer."

This prayer encounter exudes agonistic respect (Beaman 2017b; Connolly 2005), where there is a willingness to engage with the Other without desire to change that person, but instead engaging in a manner that takes equality as a given (Beaman 2017b, 98). In this spirit, Taryn was able to visit the patient without agenda or expectation, but could simply and genuinely be present. Trust was built over time, as they found the mundane common ground of a shared birthday. With the request for prayer and the comment that God was "showing up" in the hospital for this patient, any presumption of healthcare as a public, religious-free zone is made impossible; religion and prayer showed up together with the patient. Moreover, in the prayer encounter, the frame of reference shifted from caregiver and recipient of care to a mutual exchange of caring. As explained by sociologist Michael Mason (2013), who reflects on anthropologist Victor Turner's work, "Turner analysed prayer as a liminal activity, occurring in a space where participants have stripped off their everyday statuses and roles. This kind of 'nakedness' together often gives rise to an intense experience of solidarity for which Turner used the Latin term *communitas*" (21). With this posture, deep equality took form, facilitated by the prayer exchange that was replete with authenticity, affection, gratitude, and even humour.

At the beginning of this chapter, we mentioned the shifts in contexts in which hospitals are currently operating. Without question, tensions around secularism and diversity are present, but concurrently the expression of prayer and spiritual practices, the presence of chaplains, and the multi-faith spaces signal a new normal. Old dominances of majoritarian religions are falling away, now sharing space with diasporic (migrant) religions, Indigenous spiritualities, emergent spiritualities, and the non-religious. This new diversity results in power struggles and some sense of loss, but our research in London and Vancouver hospitals has provided glimpses of a reimagined, responsive, and inclusive possibility. There is a fresh excitement about trying to meet the challenge of this new diversity. A model is emerging that acknowledges difference without sliding into particularism or universalism (though traces of both remain) and that finds points of similarity rather than sameness. As put by Roshan, a Muslim administrator in London, "We come together as a group and our focus was not the differences. We come for something that is in common. We focus on the common side of things, not the differences." Within this new normal, space is created for difference, which means that in the spirit of respect, there are sites of recognition both fixed (e.g., Muslim prayer room, First Nations sacred space) and emergent through everyday interactions. Configurations and negotiations unfold within the space of difference that is created through deep equality. In the following chapter on geographies of prayer, we examine these fixed and emergent sites more closely.

Mapping Geographies of Prayer

Melania Calestani, Sonya Sharma, and Christina Beardsley

Geography matters to prayer. It matters to where, when, and why prayer can happen and how it is constructed. In this chapter we examine the mutual shaping of prayer and space, discussing formal, informal, in-between, and unexpected spaces of prayer in healthcare settings. Geographers of religion have interrogated how religion and space are co-constituted (Hopkins, Kong, and Olson 2012; Kong 2001). Similarly, literature on spiritual geographies (Bartolini et al. 2017; Henderson 1993) has presented spirituality at a range of different spatial scales; for instance, from the body to the global (Holloway and Valins 2002, 5; Bartolini et al. 2017). We build on these growing areas of research. Through mapping geographies of prayer, we observed how space, religion, and spirituality were entangled in ways that were surprising, challenging, and provocative (Bartolini, MacKian, and Pile 2018). Their entanglement revealed themes of power, inclusion, exclusion, and deep equality (Beaman 2017a). These themes highlighted how prayer could transgress clinical settings.

The concepts of map and mapping helped us to evidence and plot geographies of prayer. Maps are associated with direction and orientation, tools of representation that contain symbols, scales, and legends to graphically describe different places. They have been employed to reflect broader discourses of how the world should be seen and by whom. Additionally, maps have been used "to document and analyze socio- and psychogeographic notions of place, social relationships, and/or cognitive processes" (Powell 2010, 540). The activity of mapping enables researchers to understand subjectivities, their relation to power structures and processes of inclusions and exclusions. Here we apply the map's metaphorical powers to explore cartographies of prayer that

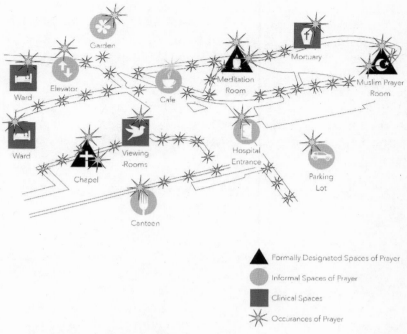

3.1 Occurrences of prayer at a hospital

were entangled with symbolism, materiality, social relations, power, and transgression of borders (Powell 2010). An integral way in which we mapped geographies of prayer was through walking interviews with our chaplain participants. Inserted above is a map of a hospital that makes visible the occurrences and social relations of prayer that chaplains discussed as we walked with them (see figure 3.1). The stars on the map indicate where prayer occurred. Prayer took place between clinical spaces (e.g., wards, mortuaries, and viewing rooms), formally designated spaces of prayer (e.g., the Muslim prayer room, the chapel, and the meditation room) and informal spaces of prayer (e.g., the canteen, the café, the hospital entrance, the parking lot, the elevator, and the corridors connecting all these different spaces). While these spaces may be read or experienced as distinct, they are not. They are fluid, in motion, never complete (Massey 2005). Theorist of religion Thomas Tweed (2006), who applies spatiality to read religious practices and spaces, similarly contends that religion is about movement and relation. The stars on the map convey religion on the move via the social relations of prayer in different spaces.

Clinical settings such as hospitals, while a stable presence in most cities and towns, are themselves spaces where people with their religious and non-religious identities and practices "cross into," "dwell" for a time, and then move on (Tweed 2006). Healthcare settings are characterized by and represent forms of change and mobility via bodies, technologies, policies, politics, and economics. Amid such dynamic clinical spaces, the lived nature of prayer is also present. We now turn to the spaces our participants showed us, mapping geographies of prayer, and providing further details on the occurrences of prayer at our field sites.

MAPPING FORMALLY DESIGNATED SPACES OF PRAYER WITHIN HEALTHCARE

As religious identities are understood as fluid (see chapter 7), so are spaces (Massey 2005). In our research we observed many different kinds of spaces within hospitals such as wards, chapels, offices, and reception areas. Because our research focused on prayer, we were particularly interested in the formally designated spaces (e.g., chapels, also referred to as sacred spaces) and the informal spaces where prayer occurred. We discovered them through our many visits to our research sites and through walking interviews with chaplains. In walking and talking with our participants, some of the formally designated spaces could be described as assigned to a religious group, inscribing fixity of religious identity and tradition onto those spaces. However, space is not an "absolute independent dimension" (Massey 1994, 3). Our observations highlighted that these spaces are "constructed out of social relations," which are "imbued with power, meaning and symbolism" (Massey 2005, 2, 3). These designated spaces were experienced and interpreted differently, depending on participants' positions on them. For example, one's gender, history, leadership role, health, or non-religious affiliation could affect participants' relations to these spaces, demonstrating that the experience of them is "constructed out of a multiplicity of social relations" that are not static and always shifting (Massey 1994, 4).

The first time we visited one London research site, we walked into the main reception area and found on a wall a directory that listed the names of each department and its location. We easily found "Chapel" and "Chaplains – Multi-faith team." In contrast, a field site in Vancouver had a more closed plan; it was not easy to find formally designated spaces of prayer, and we could not see any signs indicating how to get to these spaces. In London we proceeded to the first floor of a field site through an open foyer. On our way, we noticed art on the walls and the light, bright airy space around us. We walked along the corridor to the chaplaincy office nestled in the narthex of the chapel. The chapel was not hard to notice. It was conventionally set up with chairs in rows facing an altar that had a painting of Jesus Christ hung behind it. At the back of the chapel were a baptismal font, an organ, and a prayer request book. In the entrance to the chapel, there was a photo of the chaplaincy team, and through their clothing, one could tell that they were of different faith traditions. While the designated Christian chapel conveyed its history and tradition, it is evident that this space was not always fixed to that tradition, but other activities happened and filled this space. Christianity marked this space, but people of other faiths used it. During a walking interview, Rishi, a chaplain, told us, "During the day, lots of people come; staff come during their break and sit for some quiet time.... [E]veryone is welcome." He explained that Buddhists and Hindus often came to the chapel for prayer. Similarly, in Vancouver, when we visited a chapel at one of our sites, it was arranged with chairs in rows and a lectern and altar at the front. A prayer request book was to the back of the chapel. There was also a place for the Holy Sacrament. A chaplain described this site: "Even though you may see religious icons in the chapel, it's called a 'prayer area' or something like that. Anyone can go in." These designated spaces revealed, in different ways, that while they may seem fixed to one faith tradition, they are continually reconstituted through different bodies, beliefs, values, practices, and interactions. They are lived spaces that respond to the social relations and transformations happening around them and in which they are situated, such as the plural nature of religion and secularization.

Healthcare services have responded to religious change through the emergence of multi-faith spaces now found in other settings, such as universities and airports (Crompton and Hewson 2016; Gilliat-Ray 2005; Weller, Hooley, and Moore 2011). In one healthcare setting in Vancouver, for instance, the chapel space was created in a corner of a dining room, transforming the space from a mundane, eating space, to sacred space when folding doors were opened to reveal an altar, sacred texts, and stained-glass art. Similarly, at another site in London there was a multi-faith space, where a curtain divided the space between a Christian altar and a corner with a carpet and compass placed towards the direction of Mecca (see also chapter 2). On a walking interview, Paul (chaplain), showed us this space and described it to us: "It's a room with a curtain between two parts, and unless you actively say that's a tabernacle behind the curtain, you wouldn't actually know it's there." What was remarkable about this space was that when the curtains were pulled, it became a generic space for reflection, devoid of specific religious symbols. Somehow then, it was a fluid space that allowed it to be Christian, Muslim, or none. Scholars who have researched multi-faith spaces observe that their design does not always foster bringing faith communities together, and decorative features such as curtains can act to separate them (Eccles 2014). Like our participant implied, unless one utilizes the imaginary, they can "become like hotel rooms, approximate dwellings yet home to no one" (Crompton and Hewson 2016, 81).

At a research site in Vancouver we observed a meditation room that had a few chairs and a bookcase beneath a window. On one of the walls was a picture of a green and lush forest. Even though there was consideration given to this space, the room felt small and out of the way. On the bookcase lay a Quran and nearby on the floor was also a piece of paper under a glass pointing to Mecca. Andrew (chaplain) told us, "I get to see prayer and people going into the meditation room; Muslims use that for prayer." Despite his statement, during our fieldwork, we did not see Muslims using this room for prayer; later we were told that Muslims were more likely to pray at a nearby mosque. Multi-faith orientations that attempt to create universal spaces can often result in a lack of connection or belonging to that space (Crompton and Hewson 2016). At times the meditation room was locked because people had used it for a place to eat or nap. On a follow-up visit three months later, we realized that the piece of paper pointing to Mecca had disappeared. When we asked two of the chaplains what happened to it, they told us that it had been stolen. We were also told that the cross[1] in a meditation room was taken down, apparently without an official communication to the administration. The recent building and inhabiting of multi-faith spaces has not been easy, and at our research sites they could be a source of conflict among different faith groups and those of no affiliation, but also with management. Social anthropologist Peter Collins and colleagues (2007, 111) who conducted a study on chaplaincies in the NHS also found that such spaces were not without "contestation and negotiation." A give-and-take occurred when more than one faith group desired to access a chapel space for services. Timing, use, and the set-up of a space were aspects that required working together, and this sometimes caused tension or feeling as though one's religious tradition was being removed. Instances like these in our study signalled important power relations, but also forms of agency and working together among different user groups to ensure they had a space of their own.

In our research, walking through clinical settings with participants and listening to their stories about these different spaces raised the question of who gets space. While Muslim users can be seen to dominate multi-faith spaces because of how they are designated with curtains and carpeted floors, they can also be relegated to marginal, poorly furnished, and dimly lit rooms that are small, cramped, and without washing facilities. History, hierarchy, and power became evident in the religious and non-religious spaces found within clinical sites. The geography of religion and of prayer is inexorably linked to the politics of the built environment (Naylor and Ryan 2002). The (re)production and representation of religious landscapes always occurs within a wider contested terrain and the contingencies of other spatial processes and discursive formations (Holloway and Valins 2002), affecting architectural geographies as well as geographies of planning.

In both London and Vancouver, there was typically a historical established Christian space of prayer and other formally designated spaces. At one London site there was a small space that served those of no religious affiliation. It was minimally furnished, had a series of paintings, and shelves were erected to display sacred texts and Humanist and secular literature, signalling a space for all. However, as a result of financial constraints and lack of office space, the space was decommissioned. Although the nones are prominent in both Vancouver and London, there can be a lack of understanding as to who makes up this diverse group and their needs too for quiet, reflective, beautiful spaces. Thus, the questions of who gets space and who gets access to designated spaces were central in relation to the hierarchy of needs and the non-religious.

These questions were also relevant among minority religions. In London another site lacked a space to pray. A healthcare professional, Ersi, told us that she often advised patients to use a church nearby and that she visited it too when needed. At one point this same participant told us about a Muslim couple who needed to pray. The participant described the staff as "panicking" about what to do. Eventually a space was made for them in an office. Also, at another London site, Hindus and Sikhs questioned why they did not have a prayer space. A Hindu citizen said that she valued accommodation of minority faiths (Hinduism) but noted the uneven availability of formally designated spaces amongst religious groups. In Vancouver, Aisha, a Muslim administrator, told us they did not do prayers at work because their office was too central to the busyness of the unit, and the chapel was "too busy" with Christian symbols. Because of the lack of appropriate space, they would postpone their prayers until they got home.

We observed the instilling and crossing of spatial boundaries because of religion, non-religion, and prayer. In other words, prayer could shape the metaphorical mapping of a space or be shaped by it, as figure 3.1 also shows. Such moves revealed the contestation, politics, and agency of place-making in healthcare settings that are also viewed as public institutions. Continuing to mark designated sacred spaces and people's relationships to them are histories of power, colonialism, and hegemonic Christianity. In the next section we focus on two case studies that engage with these themes and the concept of deep equality (Beaman 2014, 2017a).

MAPPING INCLUSION AND EXCLUSION IN TWO CASE STUDIES

Walking through clinical settings revealed how inclusion and exclusion are constructed through spaces and access to them. In the two cases that follow, the intersection of race and religion symbolically marked designated spaces, mirroring what is happening in wider societies, namely the power relations affecting Indigenous people in Canada and ethnic minorities in England. These designated sacred spaces were thus sites of understanding how historical continuities of race, racism, and colonialism metaphorically map onto the social relations of prayer. The two cases have been chosen to show how power relations were embedded into formally designated spaces of prayer within healthcare settings and how prayer transgressed these processes in the negotiation of space, moving toward deep equality. We introduce the narratives of two of our participants in Vancouver and London (respectively an Indigenous elder and a chaplain) by providing some background to contextualize their words.

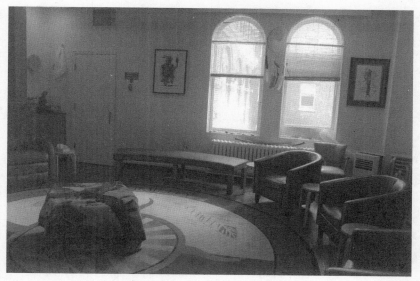

3.2 First Nations sacred space

First Nations Sacred Space

Upon walking into the First Nations sacred space in Vancouver (figure 3.2), a spirit of peace was felt. Its beauty was markedly different from the rest of the hospital, incorporating rich reds and greens, a hardwood floor, a circular carpet, and tasteful, dark, wooden shelving with Indigenous artifacts such as tea, a drum, and smudging[2] materials. Feathers, stones, and pieces of wood lined the windowsill. Indigenous art was hung on the walls and one piece depicting a mammal was entitled, "Otter – Water Spirit," a creature one might see when visiting the coastline of British Columbia. There was also a box of prayer ribbons made of red, yellow, white, and black fabric. The First Nations sacred space still represented a contact zone between European and Indigenous communities. Before it became the First Nations sacred space, it was a staff gym. During one of our visits we were told by a Euro-Canadian participant that "it used to be ours" but now it was not because it was given to the Indigenous people. In this space, healing ceremonies and prayer circles happened, especially at moments of crisis and when there was a need for rituals at the beginning or end of life.

The following story is told from excerpts of Catori's interview, an Indigenous elder. In Canada, cultural genocide happened through residential schools and the consequent removal of Indigenous children from their communities by the child welfare system. Catori told us that cultural genocide was also committed in hospitals, where Indigenous concepts of illness causation and care could not be practised. As a young child in foster care, she was forced to attend Christian church and learn various prayers. She said Psalm 23 is still important to her and she uses the imagery of "spreading a table in the presence of my enemies" as a way to move forward with respect and kindness. These are Catori's words:

We put ourselves in a circle [in the First Nations sacred space] and then we were able to spend a good couple of hours together and we shared the ceremony. And then someone else came in just to sit and read. So it affected our ability to end that. It was almost like our circle was affected. A Muslim man had come in during that time, because he was looking for a place to pray. He had his mat with him, and I guess he had done his prayer and then packed up and left. I thought that was an interesting example of how the space is designated but sometimes it's opened up beyond that.

To me the hospital administration could really look and learn about all the different sacred ways of all the people from all over the world, but especially the First Nations. Because they don't really set it [the First Nations sacred space] up to accommodate ... what the needs are. Even to have a smudge ... [talking about colonial history]. Because of the changes [the moves towards reconciliation across Canada] that are happening, I almost feel like it's redemption. That's something that was used to punish us, punish my ancestors, the Catholic church and residential schools and hospitals. They are now serving us. So, looking at it that way, it's almost "Oh, finally they let us in." ... [What feelings does the First Nations sacred space evoke in you?] That we are finally given respect. And that we have a right to be at the table. And that it saves lives ...

I truly believe that we could be further respected by having a place where we can put our items down to do the work we need to do or even refresh if we're spending time there. One day I was

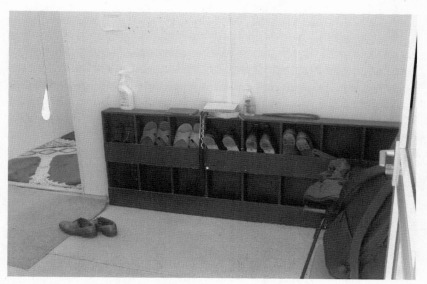

3.3 Inside a Muslim prayer room

at the hospital, before Christmas, from 9 a.m. till 9 p.m. that night. Having a place to refresh and to just relax and to store our items and debrief with each other. Having that space, I believe that we go forward, and we continue going forward, and in a respectful way, despite the treatment, despite the attitude, because somehow, somewhere it's going to happen when you continue to follow what your ancestors are guiding you to do. That respect and kindness, generosity, forgiveness go way longer than anything else.

With Catori's narrative, we heard how important the First Nations sacred space was in creating a therapeutic landscape by which this setting could be considered healing (Gesler 1992; Winchester and McGrath 2017). We were taken to this designated space by many participants during our walking interviews, and all concurred how critical the space was (see figure 3.2). As in Catori's narrative, use of the space was not without contestation, as in the case of non-Indigenous persons sharing the space. Other challenges arose when the space was not offered to Indigenous families, or when it was not accessible to them because it was locked.

Muslim Prayer Room

As global diasporic migration has brought spatial negotiation to the fore, our second case study highlights the four-year struggle at a London site to secure a permanent Muslim prayer space. The relocation of the prayer space was tied in with another project that became seriously delayed. In the later stages of the construction, the Muslim prayer room was finally relocated where male and female washing facilities were provided (see figure 3.3). It was during the period when the Muslim prayer room was unavailable that the location of Friday Prayer became an issue. The story is told from excerpts of Sophie's diary, a chaplain.

> Friday Prayer is standard in several UK hospitals. In our hospital, Friday Prayer had been accommodated in a so-called temporary clinical space. For three consecutive years it was the designated space for daily prayer during Ramadan, and in 2011 it was promised to the Multi-Faith Chaplaincy Department as the designated Muslim prayer space and a multi-faith space. However, for a period of time it became unavailable. I worked with my Muslim colleague to find an alternative venue.
>
> There was only one alternative: the lower ground floor. The space is overlooked by staircases and walkways, and the Muslim users group were concerned about the lack of privacy. They were also worried that this high visibility might lead to accusations of taking over that public space.
>
> The group asked if they could use the chapel for Friday Prayer, which had been offered under similar circumstances two years earlier and they had declined, fearing that if they did, the hospital might ignore their request for a permanent prayer space. The latter was now in sight and with no other alternative on the horizon the chapel seemed the most suitable space.
>
> As soon as the prayer space was announced on the electronic daily notice board a secretary from outpatients emailed the chaplaincy to say how distressed she was at the thought of Friday Prayer being held in the chapel. When she came to the office she prefaced her complaint with the statement "Not that I actually use the chapel myself but it's the principle." Once I explained the background and the reasons, she admitted that she admired our cooperative outlook as a chaplaincy but said that she still had reservations about what we were doing.

Friday Prayer had gone well but were tense because of conscientious objections [the Blessed Sacrament was removed] and concerns expressed by some Muslim users about entering a space with Christian images.

Over time the Muslim staff users became very skilled at setting up their temporary prayer space in various settings in the hospital on Fridays and then returning them to normal again, and this was also the case in the chapel. One colleague commented early on that it was a wonderful connective thing to have done, building a closer relationship between Muslim staff and the chaplaincy. It was symbolized by the pile of shoes outside the chaplains' office during the prayer time. In the later stages the space was finally relocated where male and female washing facilities were provided outside the prayer space.

Temporarily relocating Friday Prayer to the chapel conveyed how the negotiation of formally designated sacred spaces is indicative of power relations that amplify, enforce, and traverse perceived boundaries. Shown above, the social relations of prayer also revealed the fluidity and hybridity of these spaces. They are not fixed, but shifting because they are continually co-constituted through different bodies, beliefs, values, practices, and interactions, which can cause conflict, suspicion, resolution, and connection.

Further, healthcare contexts are public spaces "[where] diverse religious, spiritual and secularist positionalities [dwell]" (Beaumont 2008a, 6, as quoted in Kong 2010, 16). From these two case studies, we note how within these diverse spaces we make room or not for our neighbours. The cities in which the clinical sites are situated have long histories of hegemonic Christianity, colonialism, and racialization that are still present and emerge in institutional spaces. As shown above, race can mark and be read onto religious spaces and within social relations. Sociologist Les Back observes, "Racism is a spatial and territorial form of power. It aims to claim and secure territory, but it also projects associations on to space that in turn invest racial associations and attributes in places" (Back [2007] 2013, 51). Of note, "Religion is often forgotten about or is combined and subsumed under the study of race" (Hopkins 2007, 165). Nevertheless, religion is a marker for social categorization and deeply affects inclusion and exclusion in a way that is similar to race, class, gender, and age (Kong 2001). In the United Kingdom, for instance, the figure of the "Paki" has been a key object of racial hatred for several generations, and this has deeply affected post-9/11 Islamophobia in a country where most Muslims,[3] and the most recognizable Muslims, are of South Asian ancestry (Poynting and Mason 2007, 63; also see Allen 2010 and Sheridan 2006). Thus intersections of race and religion can shed light on the discourses surrounding faith groups more widely in society (Gilliat-Ray, Ali, and Pattison 2013). For example, the integration of Muslim chaplains can nurture healthcare chaplaincy reach with local constituents but simultaneously feed an agenda of securitization (Gilliat-Ray, Ali, and Pattison 2013). Likewise, Indigenous individuals and groups are given status and spaces, but these can still act to exclude them. Both case studies demonstrate how metaphorical maps of geographies of prayer need to go through several renderings for a sense of belonging to be felt. Thus inclusion and exclusion, cooperation and conflict, who gets along and who does not can be pitted as binaries that are not helpful when trying to bring together different constituents. Rather, a variation of acts, movements, and relations range between these poles and reveal deep equality at work (Beaman 2017b). When listening to and teasing out the stories of these two spaces one can discern "cooperation, agonistic respect, generosity, negotiation, forgiveness … discomfort, neighbourliness, and love" (11). In many ways and as mentioned above, most spaces we visited could be sites of both conflict and cooperation between different faith and non-faith groups and the users themselves. Where we observed less of this was in the informal spaces, where prayer showed up in areas we did not expect.

MAPPING INFORMAL SPACES OF PRAYER WITHIN HEALTHCARE

Informal spaces included unofficial sites of prayer that were in non-designated areas and identified as particularly meaningful by our participants. These were ordinary and seemingly mundane spaces (Ammerman 2007; McGuire 2008; Orsi 1985), outside of the "officially sacred" (Kong 2001). In line with sociologist of religion Sophie Gilliat-Ray's work (2010), we argue that these are spaces that are increasingly self-mediated, characterized by informal spirituality and individual sacralization.[4] For instance, some participants, like Niall and Suzanna, told us about a number of informal spaces, including a local park bench, a garden area, and an elevator that became meaningful in their mapping of the social relations of prayer: "I will pray in quiet rooms, I'll pray at a patient's bedside, I will pray out on the garden terrace. I could be comfortable praying on a garden bench in a park with a patient, if I take a patient for a walk" (Niall, chaplain, Vancouver). "We have a patio that patients can go out to. And there's been a couple of weddings there, which is great" (Suzanna, citizen, Vancouver). One might typically miss or walk by such spaces where prayer occurred, as figure 3.1 shows. Yet a canteen, parking lot, or hospital corridor became sites of prayer, reflection, and engagement with something beyond oneself. We observed that ambiguous spaces or liminal ones, using anthropologist Victor Turner's term ([1969] 2017), were constantly (re)constructed by individuals in an attempt to appropriate space and make it meaningful through prayer. These informal spaces were often transformed through the "kinetics of itinerary" (Tweed 2006) whereby religious experiences and rituals crossed and dwelled and marked space. As described in the Introduction, Frances, a chaplain, told us that a patient held up surgery, in the pre-surgery area, because he insisted he first had to have prayer. Here prayer crossed into the surgery. It became an intermediate category, bridging different categories of people, such as the clinicians and patient, and different spaces – emotional, spiritual, and clinical.

Mona, a chaplain in London, told us that, although hospitals provide designated spaces for prayer, acuity often prevents patients from accessing them. Many chaplains were more likely to pray with patients, relatives, and staff in informal spaces, such as at the bedside, or on a corridor, than in a chapel or prayer room. Religious services were celebrated regularly in hospital prayer spaces, but more people received prayer in bed during chaplain or clergy visits than at the corporate prayer itself. What was, under normal circumstances, common prayer, became individualized, and often there were pastoral and spiritual or existential needs to address before the chaplain offered the formal prayer with the patient and/or relative.

Some spaces presented challenges to chaplains when residents and patients were attached to equipment, or there was conflict and anxiety among relatives. Chaplains had to navigate physical and emotional space and also discover a metaphorical place in which to establish what was required of them at that moment. In some instances this involved leaving the bedside. Relatives were invited to continue a conversation in another room on the ward, in the long-term care space,

or in a chaplaincy office. Chaplains also spoke about learning the signals that indicated that it was time for them to leave the space.

Being able to walk with others and learn about a slice of their everyday life during walking interviews enabled us to see how chaplains
responded to their environment and how it responded to them.
Religious studies scholars Manuel Vásquez and Kim Knott (2014, 336)
note, "Religious practices like prayer are emplaced – they take place in
and creatively respond to the spatial configurations in which they are
embedded." Our participants, whom we walked with, invited us on
their trajectories, revealing how their lives and prayer were interwo-
ven in and through the healthcare settings in which they served and
worked, as depicted by the stars in the opening map (Holloway and
Valins 2002; Martin and Kryst 2005; Reimer-Kirkham et al. 2012). The
practices, spaces, and social relations of prayer by way of walking
interviews uncovered formal and informal spaces, but also in-between
and unexpected geographies of prayer, which we turn to next.

IN-BETWEEN AND UNEXPECTED

Walking has long been part of ethnographic research. It entails a
researcher's embodied participation and attunement to the social
worlds of another, grounded in shared circumstances of everyday life
for a period of time (Lee and Ingold 2006). The repeated action of
walking, one foot in front of the other, results in various routes and
paths, which enable a space to be discovered. Walking interviews, led
by participants, helped us "to understand the routes and mobilities of
others" (68). They revealed the interactions and relationships participants had with the hospital context and how the social relations of
prayer occurred in these spaces.

Walking also exposed the notion of "landscape as text" (Barnes and
Duncan 2013; Duncan 2004; Duncan and Duncan 1988), which
demonstrates how space can be read and re-read in different ways,
including reading the sacred. This is in line with geographer Lily
Kong's (2001, 2002) call to recognize the "unofficially sacred" by
including it in researchers' spatial accounts of religion (Holloway
2003). So far we have looked at formal designated spaces and the
negotiation surrounding them among different actors and informal,
ordinary, mundane spaces. We discuss informal spaces further,
explaining how they became liminal spaces, demonstrating in-
between and unexpected geographies of prayer. When we talk about

liminal spaces, we are interested in capturing the nuances that emerged when space (whether clinical, ordinary, mundane, or formally designated spaces of prayer) was appropriated by our participants in an attempt to make it relevant to their own non-religious and/or non-spiritual identities.

An example came from Julia, a Humanist chaplain, who, during a walking interview, stopped in the entrance to the chapel, which could be considered the boundary between the formally designated space of prayer and an ordinary one. With the Christian altar in the background, she gestured to a rack that displayed some Humanist booklets. This was meaningful to her, a way to make the non-religious visible in the religious space. This act could also be perceived as transgressive, crossing boundaries of official and distinct categories of spaces and producing a liminal space in-between. Julia might also be perceived as redrawing border lines of the chaplaincy by mapping a geography of the non-religious onto the space via her pamphlets, thus plotting an alternate path toward prayer and making way for inclusivity.

Another example of a geography of prayer emerged during a walking interview with Martin, a chaplain in London, who, when asked about how he defined prayer, answered, "Life is a prayer and it's our conscious contact with a God who loves us." On a Friday evening, during the walking interview, while the hospital was becoming quiet, Martin took us to where he stayed overnight when he was on duty. He then described a specific event that happened to him in a common area, which he called the "doctors' mess" (a common area for staff members). He explained how one evening he met a reconstructive burns surgeon who was going to operate on a small child who needed immediate surgery. The following day he met the mother of the child in the chapel. She came to pray and to thank God for the positive outcome of the surgery. Martin talked with her about his meeting with the surgeon and she asked him to thank the doctor on her behalf. When he summarized these events, he viewed them as being all related, "something that started in the doctors' mess, then continued in an operating room until one o'clock in the morning, and then picks up when someone comes to the chapel to give thanks before going home." He elaborated: "That's the life and being part of that interconnectedness, the whole life is a prayer, more places we go to, more life we see, the more I'm able to dwell in my understanding of what I think prayer is, to be more prayerful, being prayerful, and this is how it changes." In this story, different spaces and moments in the hospital are intertwined, proposing an unexpected geography of prayer that connects different categories of people (the chaplain, the surgeon, and the patient's mother) as well as different spaces. Ordinary and clinical spaces unexpectedly become liminal sites of prayer when prayer is enacted on the way to the operating theatre, the mortuary, or the palliative rooms, as figure 3.1 shows. Tulio, a Vancouver chaplain, said, "It was in the palliative room. That's where the church was. That's where the sacred space was; around this dying and deceased resident's bed." From this comment, we observed how prayer was brought into medical spaces, whereby the transgression of prayer in these clinical spaces resulted in their ontological remaking.

These liminal social constructions moreover can complement and conflict with biomedical meanings and applications, raising questions linked not only with deep equality (Beaman 2014, 2017a), but also with the relevance of therapeutic architecture to create spaces that include holistic concepts of care (Chrysikou 2014), such as social relations of prayer and spiritual care. The tensions between different spaces played out in hospitals cannot be reduced to binary oppositions but must take into consideration fluidity and the continual construction and deconstruction of liminal spaces. The study of prayer can therefore shed light on in-between spaces and moments that are created in healthcare, crossing and transgressing boundaries in unexpected ways, where those of faith and of no religious faith may coexist, compete at times or provide paths and bridges toward acceptance and respect. Mapping subjectivities and geographies of prayer within healthcare settings enabled us to note when liminality and transgression showed up even amidst structures of power and processes of inclusion and exclusion. The next chapter focuses on the organizational structures, values, and policies that characterized the clinical settings of our study of which a theme is how these aspects affected the institutional allocation of spaces for prayer.

4

Organizational Practices
in the Management of Prayer

Sheryl Reimer-Kirkham, Christopher De Bono, and Barry Quinn

Immediately upon entering the main entrances of hospitals in our study, one was introduced to their missions and values with, for example, a historical tribute to the religious sisters who founded the hospital or a banner listing the organization's values displayed in a spacious foyer. The question we pursue in this chapter is the extent to which this visual foregrounding of a hospital's mission statement aligns with organizational practices and everyday clinical care, and how in turn, prayer takes form in these particular settings. The expression of prayer in our research settings was sometimes explicitly visible and other times appeared as a kind of implicit hidden presence. In both the explicit and implicit expressions, however, it is our insight that prayer's visible appearance in the day-to-day is fundamentally shaped by the core priorities and values of a healthcare institution. Organizational practices can mediate transgression, to account in part for how transgressive prayer is deemed in a clinical setting.

For the sake of this comparative analysis, we have selected two of our research sites, one in London and one in Vancouver, that are roughly the same in size and the types of services provided. The sites do not necessarily represent all English and Canadian organizations, but the data gathered in these sites allows for elucidation of organizational practices that, we posit, are common. For ease and clarity, we have in this chapter given fictionalized names to these two hospitals, Oceanside Hospital in Vancouver and City Centre Hospital in London. We start by describing organizational structures, particularly in relation to mission statements and organizational leadership. Our interest is in the historical and contemporary influences that shape organizational mission statements, and how these aspirational statements are enacted. This analysis provides insight into how explicitly religious-inspired mission language compares with secular-value language. In the second section we consider resource allocation for spiritual care services and spaces as an organizational practice for the management of prayer. At Oceanside Hospital, a well-resourced spiritual care service made prayer readily visible, as well as welcome in the clinical setting. Although spiritual care services at City Centre Hospital are not resourced to the degree of the faith-based Oceanside hospital, prayer nonetheless appeared in formal and informal ways (as explained in chapter 1). In the final section we discuss findings in relation to the workplace and employees, spiritual practices and religious rituals, and making sense of suffering. While spiritual care is primarily oriented toward patients and their families, we also saw the provision of spiritual support to staff members, with evidence of staff actively engaged in spiritual practices, including prayer, while in the workplace.

These three areas – organizational mission and values; resource allocation; and employee support and expression of spirituality – fall under the umbrella of workplace spirituality. Spirituality in organizations has been described in several ways: (1) spiritual or religious practices performed in organizational settings, such as meditation or group prayer; (2) spiritual values, beliefs, or behaviours of a leader (referred to as spiritual leadership); (3) spiritual or religious values or beliefs expressed in the mission and practices of an organization; and (4) how spirituality is reflected in organizational structure and policies (Biberman and Marques 2014). We argue in this chapter that organizational practices directly and indirectly shape the expression of spirituality and prayer in healthcare settings, for good and bad (Karakas and Sarigollu 2019). As healthcare administrators (De Bono, Quinn), we bring our perspectives as insiders to the challenges of facilitating workplace spirituality in contexts of austerity and competing priorities, alongside an outsider and analyst (Reimer-Kirkham).

The chapter employs theologian Elaine Graham's seminal idea that attention to practices matters because they disclose or foreclose values in the light of changing contexts and point to the importance of practical thinking. She writes, "To ask of any practice 'What does it disclose/foreclose?' is to attempt to identify the values and preconceptions by which practices are informed. This enables a critical renewal of such values in the light of changing contexts, but honours the strategic nature of any dimension of practical reasoning" (2002, 163). Graham explains that disclosive practices illuminate inclusive strategies and policies, in contrast to foreclosive practices that gloss over relations of power with insistence upon universalist and essentialist models of human nature (9). The heuristic contribution of this dialectal question, "What does it disclose/foreclose?" to our analysis of prayer lies in its ability to look behind common organizational practices (and our own vantage points) in a reflexive, responsible way. We employ this dialectic throughout the chapter, considering organizational practices that disclose (i.e., illuminate or hold space for spirituality and prayer) or foreclose (i.e., obfuscate or deny space for spirituality and prayer).

MISSION STATEMENTS AND ORGANIZATIONAL LEADERSHIP: "REALIZING A PHILOSOPHY"

The challenge facing any healthcare organization is to articulate its unique mission and values and to operationalize them through its leaders, resource allocation, human resource management, and everyday clinical care. One might expect that when it comes to spiritual care services (and prayer), this articulation and operationalization might be relatively explicit in a faith-based organization such as Oceanside Hospital, and more implicit or even lacking in a secular organization such as City Centre in London. However, our extended fieldwork and careful analysis of the situated practices at each site have revealed a more complex picture. In both settings there are openings or opportunities in the organizational mission statements and values that allow for (disclose) meeting the needs of religious diversity, the integration of spiritual care, and a responsive person-centredness vis-à-vis personal values, beliefs, and practices, including prayer. And, as explained in this chapter, in both settings there are competing practices that can at times foreclose on spirituality.

Historically both Vancouver and London research sites have religious ties, thanks to the pioneering work of religious sisters in the former, and the longstanding Christian influence in the latter. What is different is that Oceanside remains an independent religiously sponsored hospital financed almost entirely by a government-owned health authority, while City Centre is owned and operated by the National Health Service (NHS), where the NHS is itself differentiated from the Church of England (Eccles 2014).

Mission Statements and Values

Oceanside Hospital explicitly presents itself as being mission and vision driven so as to create patient experiences for all, without prejudice, that reflect compassionate caring and social justice. Its mission statement explicitly uses religious language and identifies spiritual needs as part of the care the organization is dedicated to providing. At the core of its mission work are values that combine socio-religious teaching and ecumenical references (e.g., to God and Jesus Christ) with values-language (e.g., trust, respect, dignity). Its challenge is to retain the historical Christian identity mandated by its owners and bylaws in a way that remains universal; that is, to create an inclusive ethos for patients and employees, caring for those who identify as religious and non-religious.

City Centre Hospital, part of the NHS, recently conducted a consultation with staff, users, and the local population to develop a set of values or mission ethos. The values reflect the current NHS priority to develop services focused on person-centred care. Central to these values is striving to be attentive, respectful, and responsive to the diverse needs (physical, social, emotional, and spiritual) of those who use the services and the staff who help deliver them. Thus City Centre's values-orientation creates space for the integration of spiritual care and prayer. As an example of how the values might be operationalized to encompass spirituality in an inclusive spirit, Elaine, an administrator, reflected on a talk she gave: "The culture of 'unfailing kindness,' I don't know whether you would describe that as spiritual or not, but the culture of being welcoming and hospitable to patients is probably one of the most important things in the delivery of healthcare. Religion for some people will be really important and for others it will be less important. But I don't know anybody who doesn't want the people who are looking after them to be really kind to them." It is not clear whether this administrator was explicitly aware that she was connecting the historic link between hospitality and hospital (Connell and Beardsley 2014; Pesut et al. 2012), but she underscores a core spiritual value in her appeal to kindness. This tension between whether explicit religious language or spiritual reference needs to be used in mission statements, or even ought to be used, surfaced in the study. For example, there was inconsistency among participants' perceptions at City Centre Hospital about whether spiritual expression (beyond the services of chaplaincy) was freely allowed. In this way, the concept or practice of spirituality could come down to people and their particular propensities, a finding we have reported at other Canadian sites (Reimer-Kirkham and Cochrane 2016; Reimer-Kirkham et al. 2018), and an approach that forecloses (or does not recognize) organizational spirituality.

Organizational experts are well aware of the possible gap between the ideal of a mission and vision, and their operationalization. Organizational expert Edgar Schein (2010, 28) says, "Consensus on the core mission and identity does not automatically guarantee that the key members of the organization will have common goals or that the various subcultures will appropriately align to fulfil the mission." Additionally, as Mona put it, operationalization depends on intentional monitoring and structure: "They have this in the mission statement that they look after you. How much of it is followed up? Mission statements are nice things and make the organization look good, but I don't know how often they revisit it to see how well we're achieving anything" (chaplain, London). This comment captures the heart of the matter: are organizations able to translate high ideals into practical care? Tracing this idea of realizing a philosophy or mission, we describe leadership structures and philosophies at the two sites.

Organizational Leadership Structure and Philosophy

The organizations have embedded their commitment to their mission and values into their leadership structures in a variety of ways. City Centre Hospital relies primarily on people to carry the mission forward, whereas Oceanside Hospital has a more formalized approach with a dedicated portfolio that is structured to support its people in living the mission and values. Laura, an administrator, commented on the distinctiveness of Oceanside as a faith-based provider: "What does it mean to be a religiously affiliated hospital in a secularized context? It makes it very challenging [*laughs*]. But it is what has allowed us to stay separate when health authority structures came together." Two decades ago, government restructured health services so that over 200 separate hospitals, each with its own board and historical identity, were merged into five health authorities. The one exception was that twenty-one faith-based organizations, with Oceanside Hospital among them, through an agreement with the government were able to maintain their faith-based identity in such a way that they could "own and operate" their facilities to reflect their mission.

Oceanside Hospital embeds its mission and values across its leadership. The bylaws require that all members of the board of directors and society that governs the board subscribe to the religiously inspired mission of the organization. Senior leaders must also do so. Laura reflected on the importance of "having a position at the senior team whose role is to keep mission and values integrated in the organization and make sure we're being true to our ethical framework." Additional (and related) organizational structures ensure the enactment of the religiously inspired mission: (1) at the governance level of the board, a subcommittee of directors form the Mission and Ethics Committee, which is accountable to the board for issues relevant to mission integration; (2), a Mission, Values, and Ethical Framework is embedded in the strategic plan; and (3) a mission formation program to equip each level of staff extends from an orientation workshop for all new staff to an extended residential program for senior leaders. With these leadership structures and philosophy, Oceanside Hospital is intentional in creating and communicating a culture that integrates its healing mission into operational leadership and clinical care. A question we will return to is how such top-down, organizationally driven integration creates space for prayer.

In London the leadership and management at City Centre Hospital reflect local engagement with its values as well as the principles of the NHS as a whole; indeed, all staff are expected to share the hospital and NHS vision. In this way the operationalization of the City Centre's mission and values occurs through people, perhaps more so than structures or programs. Thus the degree to which leaders recognize their own leadership role can shape the operationalization of the mission and values to include the support for spiritual care and prayer. This was reflected on by a participant in London:

> RESEARCHER: And what about the organizational mission and the values of this hospital? Do you think that their organizational mission and values include the support for spiritual care, for prayer?
> MARGARET: Oh well, they seem to. I've met the chief nurse who seems pro, and the chief executive seems pro, and the chairman of the board seems pro. What would happen if they weren't? I don't

know. Because my suspicion is that it's more to do with personalities than it should be.

As at Oceanside Hospital, attention is put to leadership development in the NHS. Recent work by the NHS Leadership Academy has encouraged leaders and managers to consider the role of "partnership leadership" linked to servant leadership as described by Greenleaf (2002). This leadership style is focused on the growth and well-being of others and the community, team, or organization. The approach moves the leader or senior team from a place of power to one of engaging with others as the "servant" and/or "partner." It is hoped that this bottom-up approach may lead to increased staff engagement and retention and to providing person-centred care and improved job satisfaction (Quinn 2017).

To summarize, thus far we have seen how spiritual care (and prayer) are explicitly supported at executive and organizational levels at Oceanside Hospital, with structures and leadership philosophies to equip and embed a distinctive religious identity and values throughout the organization. City Centre Hospital takes a different approach to organizational culture that is values-informed, dependent upon individuals at all levels of the organization to live out the values. An emphasis on leadership development, specifically servant leadership, equips leaders to do so. Moving from the overarching level of mission and values, through organizational structures and leadership philosophy, we next explore how research allocation makes invisible and visible organizational priorities for spiritual care and prayer.

RESOURCES FOR SPIRITUAL CARE AND PRAYER: "PUTTING OUR MONEY WHERE OUR MOUTH IS"

Schein (2010, 236) presents embedding mechanisms as "major 'tools' that leaders have available to them to teach their organizations how to perceive, think, feel and behave based on their own conscious and unconscious convictions." One of these embedding mechanisms is how leaders allocate resources, while another is the design of physical space, facades, and buildings. The challenging decision of how to allocate resources continues to be made against changing priorities in health and social care need and limited resources. Whereas both of our sites found ways to resource chaplaincy services and sacred spaces, other organizations have not held onto this priority. For example, in chapter 5 we reference other healthcare organizations in Canada that have disbanded their spiritual care departments, and we were recently told of a sacred space in another city that was used for storage of medical equipment. In the following section we look first at resource allocation (human resources) for spiritual care and then spatial resource allocation (designated sacred spaces) as disclosing and foreclosing prayer at Oceanside Hospital and City Centre Hospital.

Allocation of Human Resources for Spiritual Care

Chaplaincy services at Oceanside strive, according to its senior leader, to be a leading best practice clinical and organizational department, which seeks to make concrete the relationship between spirituality, religion, and health. This department links its work directly to the organization's vision as a ministry of compassion to all patients, residents, their families, and to the leaders, staff, and volunteers. Similarly tracing a line between who an organization says it is (its mission statement) and the allocation of resources for spiritual care, Laura put it this way: "First of all, it's putting our money where our mouth is. Almost every organization in healthcare somehow in their mission statement talks about holistic care. And yet, how can you have holistic care and not provide resources for the spiritual side that is part of holistic care?... We would fight tooth and nail if there was ever any kind of pushback from our funders about where we're allocating our resources for spiritual care." These comments made by the department and Laura revealed tensions about resource allocation. Oceanside far out-staffs its secular Canadian counterparts, both regionally and nationally. The number of chaplains here, funded from the hospital's operating budget, is roughly one chaplain per 100 patients/residents, a number reported as near or above the provincial and national average.[1] Participants at this site recognized that this level of resourcing for spiritual care communicates organizational affirmation of prayer: "Certainly, they're employing a staff as big as the spiritual care department is a huge way of advocating for prayer and spiritual practices. This is quite extraordinary for them, for there to be as many chaplains as there are. Them putting their money where their values are is pretty big" (Niall, chaplain, Vancouver). A strength of this well-resourced model is the visible presence of spiritual care. This resourcing discloses organizational support for spirituality to be treated as a clinical variable, to be included and addressed as part of interdisciplinary care.

Angela, an administrator, confirmed the presence of chaplains: "I go to clinical rounds on some teams. There's always a chaplain there." However, a weakness of the model is the constitution and resourcing of those in chaplain roles. There is a certain foreclosure in the composition (representation) of the chaplaincy team. While they are trained to assess and respond to all spiritual care needs, including those outside their own tradition, the particular traditions reflected in the current staffing are mainly Christian-affiliated.

Tensions were identified in care provided to Indigenous peoples. Indigenous spiritual care has traditionally not been resourced under the umbrella of Oceanside's spiritual care services but instead has been managed by an Indigenous Wellness team.[2] This split structure was flagged by Catori, an Indigenous elder: "All these spiritual care providers are on salary paid full-time with full benefits. What they give us elders is a piddly honorarium for the huge work that we do, sometimes seven days a week. It's ridiculous, and very, very unacceptable." In the era when all Canadian organizations and citizens are called to take up the recommendations of the Truth and Reconciliation Commission of Canada (2015),[3] there is a clear mandate to respond to the diverse population served. A recent organizational realignment has allowed for closer integration of Indigenous services with spiritual care services, disclosing a new openness toward culturally responsive, equitable care for Indigenous peoples.

Responsiveness to the population served was also a key consideration at City Centre Hospital where Britain's 2012 Health and Social Care (Safety and Quality) Act and the 2006 and 2010 Equality Acts form a legislative structure that requires care of patients whatever their religion or belief (NHS 2015 Chaplaincy Guidelines). The 2015 NHS Chaplaincy Guidelines (NHS 2015) advise an allocation of hours per week of chaplaincy care based on the number of patients and staff, with posts matched by religion or belief, including care for those "not identified with a particular faith or belief system." While these guidelines disclose a human rights–informed sensitivity to ensuring a diverse chaplaincy staff that mirrors the population, the challenge comes in that these are only guidelines. As a result, resource allocation for spiritual care is made in relation to other priorities in the hospital. Research into funding and resource allocation for all services across the NHS indicates that the funding challenges for chaplaincy are part of a much bigger funding crisis (Robertson et al. 2017). John, an administrator, explained: "It's getting harder and harder for [these spiritual and religious] resources, especially in terms of funding. It's always going to be what are the other priorities in the hospital. But at the moment, although the resources are really tight, it is maintaining the service. I can say that it's not enough, it could be more. I can't add any more to what is already stretched, and I'm at the point now when I'll be recruiting two or three people to join the team because we've lost those, it's going to be quite tricky to hold the balance between how much you get to pay for them, and how much is available." A 2013 BBC report on chaplaincy in the NHS revealed the number of staff employed on the chaplaincy team at City Centre as slightly below the national average. The chaplaincy staffing at this site is also below the NHS guidelines (2015, 16) and one-quarter of the Ocean-side Hospital allocation (even though the patients served is roughly equivalent). As a result, much of the spiritual care support offered to patients, family, and staff is delivered by a large number of chaplaincy volunteers. Connor told us, "I would have said out of our hospital budget, we don't invest a lot in chaplaincy. I think for every one chaplain we pay, we probably have about three or four or five volunteer chaplains. And if we just got what we paid for, it would be very low. So yes, we don't really invest in chaplains" (administrator, London). These figures give insight into priorities and making difficult decisions about limited resources and increasing demands. Similar to most NHS Trusts (and the Canadian sites), the majority of employed chaplaincy staff come from a Christian background, with one part-time staff member from a Muslim background. The volunteers represented a much more diverse group. Via the embedding mechanism (Schein 2010) of resource allocation for spiritual care, City Centre Hospital seemed to foreclose support for prayer; in other words, with fewer chaplains to offer prayer, these needs may be missed. This foreclosure is offset by the embedding mechanism of investing in physical space, facades, and buildings, where City Centre's design communicates a centrality of religious and spiritual plurality and discloses or makes visible spiritual practices in healthcare settings.

Allocation of Spatial Resources

Discussed in more detail in chapter 3, the spatial allotment for designated sacred spaces at each of the research sites communicated significant value placed on organizationally supporting spirituality in the workplace. Interestingly, in our comparator hospitals, formal space allocation for designated sacred spaces is similar. If faith-based organizations do this from an explicitly religious motivation, we wondered why secular hospitals might do it. It appears that social trends (and corresponding legislation as earlier noted), such as migration and the need to accommodate staffs' own religious needs, are motivating factors.

At City Centre Hospital, the formally designated spaces held a prominent place in the architectural layout, with a Christian chapel (accommodating twenty-five to thirty attendees), a Muslim prayer room (accommodating fifty attendees), and a garden area, all situated in an expansive centre foyer. Much of the public space is bright, containing art intended to promote a calming, healing atmosphere. Reflecting population trends in both patients and staff, and like many other hospitals in London, this site now makes room for those from the Muslim traditions: "As a Muslim community, prayer is one of our main pillars of religion, and that's why we always try to get a space for our people, because all Muslim people, wherever they live, need to pray" (Roshan, administrator). Thus the allotment of space disclosed a welcoming stance toward prayer and related spiritual practices that occur in designated sacred spaces. As a counterpoint, one could question whether there was an element of containing religion to these spaces – though this argument does not hold well as religion spilled out into the clinical areas of the hospital, such as when chaplains and volunteers visited in their clerical collars and religious garb (Crompton and Hewson 2016). Also, as counterpoint, though sacred spaces were centrally and prominently located at our London sites, participants had their own preferences for which sacred space was more conducive to prayer. For example, Paul (chaplain) preferred the Christian chapel, where he could reflect on a painting of Jesus Christ.

At Oceanside Hospital in Vancouver, the chapel is hard to find, away from the main entrance and the clinical areas. It has a low ceiling and a rectangular shape, and accommodates up to thirty-five people. In the original building the chapel was larger, with soaring ceilings, and centrally located, but with renovations to accommodate additional clinical space, the chapel was eventually relocated. Something similar happened with the newer First Nations sacred space. While innovative and nicely decorated inside, it too is located out of the way. Patient or visitor access to this space required a member of the Indigenous Wellness team, which meant it was not easily accessible for a drop-in visit. The gardens also emerged as an important informal sacred space.

Overall there was considerable variation at the research sites in the visibility and space allocation of the designated spiritual spaces. In some sites, the welcoming, aesthetic public spaces lent to spiritual reflection and centrally located formal sacred spaces (whether a Christian chapel, a Muslim prayer room, or a multi-faith space, as described in chapters 2 and 3) disclosed support for prayer. In those sites where the visibility and space allocation were low, the effect was to dissuade or foreclose (Graham 2002) easy access to (formal) prayer, and in the case of Oceanside, implicitly contradict the overt, religious organizational mission.

ORGANIZATIONAL PRACTICES AND EMPLOYEES' WORKPLACE SPIRITUALITY: "PERMISSION TO PRAY"

In this last section we explore organizational practices in workplace spirituality and how prayer takes form for and with staff. A more direct observance of organizational practices for the management of prayer was how staff were allowed or supported to engage in prayer if they so desired. It was not unusual to see staff praying in designated sacred spaces during our fieldwork. One of the nurses we interviewed in Vancouver, for example, said he attended Mass every day, as did staff in London for Friday Prayer in Muslim prayer rooms: "You can see people coming just like that, with the scrubs. They have just a small time to come and pray. Ten minutes, fifteen minutes. They turn up in their scrubs. They do it" (Roshan, administrator). Meditative practices (mindfulness) were offered weekly at one Vancouver long-term care facility, and several leaders at religiously affiliated sites mentioned the practice of prayer or meditation at the beginning of meetings.

However, other participants in both London and Vancouver were reticent about the appropriateness of saying prayers as employees at work. A manager in Vancouver did not feel she had a place conducive to say her Muslim prayers, so she would instead invite staff to go on a short meditative walk. An administrator in London mused, "What about this environment gives me permission to pray, whatever that means for me? And that's for staff and patients. I don't think this environment gives people permission to transgress, to break the rules, to pray. What would that look like?" (Connor). At the level of staff engaging in prayer, then, there was considerable variation.

At our research sites another dimension of staff spirituality was disclosed: spiritual support to staff. The chaplaincy teams were clear they provided spiritual support to staff; structurally, the job descriptions at both organizations permitted staff spiritual support. Our interviews offered interesting insights into how spirituality transcends or adds to the context, even when resourcing for available support is thin. In London, Connor went on to say, "I love spending time with them [chaplaincy team] because they're beyond the medical, but I think they only reach a fraction of the staff. I think there's something about supporting the staff for the staff to support the patient." This insight into the way spirituality can assist with trends towards the over-medicalization of healthcare was confirmed by another case where staff asked a chaplain for a way to ritually move through the suffering they felt after the death of homeless person in their care. "They were very touched by that suffering and they asked me, 'Would you please release the soul of this person?' They don't learn about soul in medical school and they ask me, 'Please release the soul. Do something to dignify this person.' The medical community sometimes needs some prayer rituals to help them process the grief and to create some sort of healing environment, like accepting the mystery of death and dying or suffering. To ritualize human life, to give some dignity by ritualizing, saying goodbye to somebody" (Andreas, chaplain, Vancouver). This theme of chaplaincy offering a balancing, humanizing resource was recurrent. At times it revealed a tension in resourcing. An administrator said, "If you said to me, would I rather have a critical care outreach nurse or a chaplain, you're going to get a different answer. And at the moment I haven't got enough critical care outreach nurses" (Stanley). In the same interview, he acknowledged the reality of the chaplain supporting patients, families, and the clinical team at times of great suffering. The administrator recalled his own example of the night when a young mother died shortly after giving birth, and the impact this had on him and the team. "When people die, there isn't more of a failure than that. And when a young woman dies in the process of giving birth, can you think of anything worse? So yes, blame and guilt and shame and all those kinds of things and of course all the professional groups are looking at one another, wondering who did it." In this example, the participant understood that staff members are exposed to the suffering of another and they must find a way of making sense of what they witness. He went on to describe the comforting and – in this situation – the necessary presence of the chaplain, and the role of ritual for all who were present. "This was really hard in head space and heart space. Forget all the other stuff going on. And he [the chaplain] held everybody in the team. Very calm. And there was a whole lot of religious ritual that he brought to it, which was very comforting. It was another dimension that he brought to that with a whole set of rituals that could be followed. And I think people found that very helpful. And he orchestrated that. He brought it all together." This example reveals the visible and invisible presence of suffering that is an everyday part of these hospitals, the impact on the staff members who witness it, and the supportive presence of the chaplain. Although pain and suffering are in some ways synonymous in the contemporary culture, physician Eric Cassell (1998) suggests that they are quite distinct. While pain can be experienced on many levels, suffering arises from the meaning individuals make of the experience of that pain or the apparent meaninglessness of what they are facing. The suffering, the meaningless, or the spiritual distress that Cassell refers to may be invisible at times, yet it assumes a very real presence within healthcare contexts and staff members encounter it regularly (Quinn 2012). These stories of prayer and support by and for staff as part of meaning-making in the face of suffering suggest, in our view, the very real value and support for prayer and ritual within healthcare organizations.

To conclude, there are challenges and cautions in the variety of organizational approaches to supporting spirituality and prayer. This study pointed to convergences and differences in the ways that a religiously affiliated organization compares with a secular one. We have traced Graham's (2002) disclosure/foreclosure dialectic through mission/values statements to organizational structures and leadership philosophy to resource allocation to clinical integration to employee workplace support to reveal how space is held for prayer, and in turn, how religion and spirituality are integrated into healthcare settings. This angle of analysis helps to account for why and how prayer is deemed transgressive in many situations (as recounted in other chapters). Whether an organization holds an explicit religious mission that is patient-focused or whether an organization communicates values such as person-centredness, respect, inclusion, and kindness, an interpretation of this as allowing prayer can be foreclosed or negated by other organizational practices such as reduced resource allocation for chaplains (as at City Centre Hospital) or hard-to-find or hidden designated sacred spaces (as at Oceanside Hospital). Our analysis here shows the complexity and idealism of seeking coherence across an organization. In some situations, it truly "comes down to the person," but our research also showed that broader, organizationally structured approaches can influence the way prayer appears in healthcare contexts. So, while prayer may not easily fit into competing organizational and clinical priorities, an organization can message the degree to which holistic and person-centred care can hold space for prayer, and how spirit at work can offset the suffering healthcare workers witness and endure. Chaplaincy, the focus of the next chapter, is a primary mechanism for such messaging.

Chaplaincy in Canada and the United Kingdom: Prayer and the Dynamics of Spiritual Care

Christina Beardsley, Andrew Todd, and Sheryl Reimer-Kirkham

"Nurses and physicians can do a spiritual screening, but I don't know that they can really do an adequate assessment. That's that piece about valuing spirituality in the whole system, and if you don't value spirituality you're not going to value prayer. You're only going to see prayer as an external action, not as something that is deeply rooted, connected, and has impact on one's hospital experience and health outcomes."[1]

Curtis, chaplain, Vancouver

These comments by Curtis get at the heart of the dynamics of prayer and spiritual care in hospital contexts, with explicit focus on the unique role of spiritual care and chaplaincy services. This chapter contextualizes the research on prayer in public healthcare in relation to spiritual care in Canada and the United Kingdom.[2] Our primary interest is how chaplaincy, despite the specific nature of the research sites, is located and negotiated in public healthcare in the two countries. This contextualization is designed to explore the interplay between chaplaincy practice and how prayer is accommodated and resisted in healthcare settings. The chapter begins with brief histories of the development of chaplaincy in each setting. The next section introduces a diagrammatic conception of spiritual care in hospital to provide background to current practices and challenges. Finally, the chapter considers the liminality of chaplaincy, an important, albeit demanding feature of spiritual care; and in particular how the liminality of prayer itself intersects with the liminality of the chaplain's membership on multidisciplinary teams, such as clinical rounds, care conferences, and ethics consultations. With chaplaincy holding this liminal space in hospitals, in some circumstances there could be an element of surprise and a sense of transgression when prayer occurred.

THE HISTORICAL DEVELOPMENT OF CHAPLAINCY

The long, evolving history of spiritual care in Canada and the United Kingdom shares some commonalities, but also reflects differences. In Canada the development of chaplaincy begins in the 1600s with the establishment of hospitals by religious orders associated with European colonial expansion; Catholic with French settlers, or Anglican with British settlers. Religious and spiritual care as now understood previously belonged to church-funded health services provided or administered mainly by religious sisters, and to a lesser degree by religious brothers and priests. Religious health service delivery continued for several centuries, until the post–Second World War establishment of a public welfare system that included healthcare. The history of some of our Vancouver research sites mirrors this trajectory, with religious orders travelling from Eastern and Central Canada in the late 1800s to found hospitals and care homes in Western Canada. With federal government funding that accompanied the Hospital and Diagnostic Services Act (passed in 1957) and the Medical Care Act (passed in 1966), healthcare was increasingly consolidated into regions with centralized governance. Many hospitals previously administered by religious organizations became "secular" in their governance. Today 5 per cent of Canada's healthcare is provided by faith-based organizations (Hoskins 2017). Canada's transformation away from religious organizations providing hospital services coincided with the development of chaplaincy.

The professionalization of chaplaincy in Canada has its roots in the United States in the 1920s (King 2007). Anton Boisen, a hospital chaplain influenced by Drs Cabot and Worcester of Harvard Medical School and Episcopal Theological Seminary, conducted the first program of what would become Clinical Pastoral Education (CPE) in Massachusetts in 1925 (Jernigan 2002), bringing together clinical experience with theological study. Boisen's clinical theology method tested the conceptual content of religious beliefs against human experience (deVelder 1994, 283). From the late 1930s the CPE movement attracted students from Canada (Stokoe 1974), who returned to take up Canadian hospital chaplaincy positions (sometimes sponsored by denominations or churches). CPE was being delivered in Canadian centres by the early 1950s; British Columbia's first CPE program was established in 1967. A national organization of supervised pastoral education was formed in 1965, first under the title Canadian Council for Supervised Education, renamed as Canadian Association for Pastoral Education (CAPE/ACEP) in 1974, and subsequently in 2010 as Canadian Association for Spiritual Care (CASC/ACSS) (CASC n.d.). Canada's relatively ecumenical and irenic religious scene eased the coalition of CPE centres into a national organization. Most Canadian CPE sites retain affiliation with theological schools, although the latest change in nomenclature suggests a philosophical shift from "ministry" and "pastoral" to "clinical" and "spiritual" (De Bono 2012). The-ologian and chaplain Christopher De Bono (16) notes that many Canadian chaplains are "distancing themselves from their theological, religious and ecclesial roots, often embracing more existential, entirely immanent and otherwise non-theistic approaches to practice." As explained below, the professionalization of chaplaincy has taken a somewhat different route in Britain, and yet the dynamics at our research sites were remarkably similar.

Prior to the UK welfare state, the poor were sent to parish work-houses, and associations of poverty and incarceration clung to public hospitals opened on workhouse infirmary sites long after the NHS was founded in 1948. The London sites reflect this history of voluntary hospitals and workhouse infirmaries. One of our hospitals in London was founded as a free hospital for "relieving the sick and needy," supported by private subscriptions (Humble and Hansell 1974, 12). At another of our sites, the previous building had been a workhouse infirmary. Both kinds of institution are considered formative in the very early modern professionalization of chaplains (Swift 2009, 29–40).

There were only approximately twenty-eight full-time hospital chaplains nationally in 1948. A 1951 commission on hospital chaplains marked the dawn of professional chaplaincy, and the foundation of the Hospital Chaplaincies Council (HCC), though at this date chaplains were normally expected to return to parish ministry (Swift 2009, 41). A former voluntary hospital, with its medical and nursing schools,

City Centre Hospital (one of our research sites, named in chapter 4) moved sites several times, but in close proximity to the Houses of Parliament and Westminster Abbey, whose clergy often served as its chaplains. Part-time chaplaincy continues in some hospitals, but the main change that accompanied the founding of the NHS was that chaplains were directly employed by the service rather than by their religious bodies. Thus the NHS began to shape chaplaincy, and from the late 1950s onward publications appeared exploring chaplains' professional identity in healthcare. Although mainly opinion-based, with a paternalistic, Christian focus (Swift 2009, 46), authors like theologian and chaplain Norman Autton and theologian J.G Cox, along with later writers like Michael Wilson in the 1970s and Peter Speck (whose 1988 book *Being There* distinguished between religious and spiritual care) are considered pioneers of a contemporary model of UK healthcare chaplaincy, increasingly shaped by a growing knowledge base, shared practice, and professional standards.

What had been a gradual professionalization of UK healthcare chaplaincy suddenly gathered speed from the late 1990s and in the early twenty-first century. Key factors include research into Britain's changing religious demographic and the momentum towards multi-faith chaplaincy; the impact of data protection legislation; the modernization agenda pursued by the New Labour Government, including Department of Health initiatives on healthcare chaplaincy (DOH 2003); growing academic interest in spirituality in healthcare; increasing collaboration between the UK chaplaincy bodies, including their largely successful struggle to replace the faith-mandated notion of chaplaincy favoured by HCC (now no more) with a healthcare professional model upheld by the standardizing of continuing professional development through the UK Board of Healthcare Chaplaincy (UKBHC); and the development of post-graduate degrees in chaplaincy and related studies. Chaplaincy studies scholar Christopher Swift (2009) provides a detailed account of these developments; further background and their local impact on the London sites is described in the following section.

CONTEMPORARY DYNAMICS OF CHAPLAINCY

Chaplaincy has evolved to become "a practice of care involving the intentional recognition and articulation of the sacred by nominated individuals authorized for this task in secular situations" (Swift,

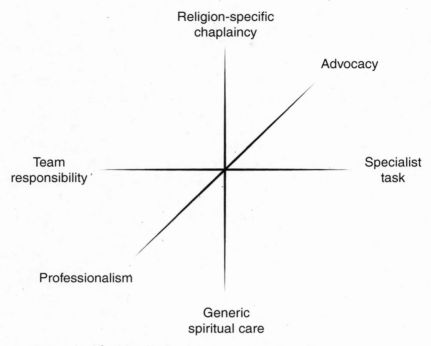

5.1 Dynamics of spiritual care

Cobb, and Todd 2015, 2). These authors stress that this type of care is a practical and relational discipline, requiring an ability to understand and take responsibility for meeting some or all of the spiritual needs of the person being cared for. This relational quality of chaplaincy is strongly reflected in our study. Chaplains work in chaplaincy teams, as members of multidisciplinary teams with responsibilities for the spiritual and religious needs of those in their care. Chaplains also have overlapping responsibilities to their institutions, providing spiritual care to staff as part of their job description. Many chaplains are also endorsed by their own faith communities, and this endorsement, which is a kind of sponsorship, carries additional relational accountabilities. These complex, overlapping domains, with their shifting boundaries, are the locus for the patterns of chaplaincy's relational practice. To visualize this relationality, and as a prelude to what follows, figure 5.1 offers a snapshot of the key dimensions around which chaplaincy care is located and negotiated. Developed in the context of this study, the diagram is also rooted in our respective knowledge as a chaplain (Beardsley), chaplaincy studies academic (Todd), and academic healthcare researcher (Reimer-Kirkham) of Canadian and UK chaplaincy.

Religion-Specific Chaplaincy or Generic Spiritual Care

The dynamic portrayed in the diagram's vertical axis depicts the extent to which spiritual care is a generic practice or a religion-specific practice, and here we see the definitional tension between religion and spirituality at work (introduced in the Introduction). If generic chaplaincy is concerned with the patient's "search for meaning ... irrespective of their religion or their philosophy of life" (Zock 2008, 137, as quoted in De Bono 2012, 194), what distinguishes such existential counselling from that of other therapists in the healthcare team? If, on the other hand, a chaplaincy service is mainly religious, and therefore mainly for one group of patients, why should public health fund it? The distinction between spiritual and religious care is well established in healthcare chaplaincy, and in both countries chaplains' attempts to broaden their professional appeal by attending to spiritual rather than religious needs, and thereby connecting with those who identify as non-religious, have mirrored societal shifts from organized religion to spirituality and non-religion (Woodhead 2016).

As Curtis noted, "There are two schools of thought ... one tends to match the spiritual tradition of the person with the spiritual tradition of the care provider. I much prefer the model where it's a multi-faith approach." Curtis's choice of the word *multi-faith* requires important contextual interpretation. In many countries, including Canada, multi-faith chaplaincy is understood generically as being "interfaith" rather than "faith-specific" (see Liefbroer et al. 2017, 1777), whereas the UK multi-faith chaplaincy model tends to be religion-specific. Sociologist of religion Sophie Gilliat-Ray and chaplain Mohammed Arshad (2015) define this UK model as the inclusion of chaplains from a range of faith communities to oversee the religious needs of those of their faith community. They note the importance of teamwork in making this work and how chaplains of different faiths can and do, in fact, substitute for one another (which begins to move toward the generic model).

UK legislation, and equal opportunities and diversity policies, are political drivers that have significantly shaped recent chaplaincy care policy in England (NHS England 2015) and Scotland (NHS Scotland

2007). Such explicit attention to equality has not been apparent in the Canadian chaplaincy discourse or policy. However, the current focus on spiritual care for Indigenous patients and families, which acknowledges their social suffering in residential schools, many of which were administered by religious organizations, has led some chaplaincies to incorporate vented rooms as sacred spaces, to facilitate ceremonial practices like smudging (see chapter 3).

Alternatively, negotiation on the diagram's religion-specific chaplaincy or generic spiritual care axis may focus on titles. In Canada (and the United States), the current nomenclature is "spiritual care practitioner" (Handzo et al. 2014, 44); in British Columbia, the title transitioned to "spiritual health practitioner" several years ago. More recently, "pastoral care" has been reintroduced in some sites. Taryn, a Vancouver chaplain, explained that she found the term "'spiritual health practitioner' unhelpful ... in crisis situations" when she reverted "to our former term 'pastoral care.'" In the United Kingdom, for some, "chaplain" has transcended its Christian roots and applies to other religious traditions, giving rise to Muslim chaplaincy (Gilliat-Ray, Ali, and Pattison 2013), for example. For others (Robinson, Kendrick, and Brown 2003, 9), and more recently for Humanists, the term *chaplain* is problematic, implying that chaplains are subject to their religious institution and unable to deliver patient-centred care.

In relation to the definition of chaplaincy cited above (Swift, Cobb, and Todd 2015, 2), this negotiation signals the value of the word *sacred*, which can encompass religious concepts of a supernatural realm, various ideas of spirituality, humanistic belief in the dignity of human life, or the little understood values and beliefs of the growing number of nones or those who identify as having no religion. That spiritual care encompasses the sacred also highlights some of chaplaincy's dilemmas in a pluralistic setting. Curtis spoke "of a potentially spiritual crisis in the grand culture." For example, handling worship, liturgy, and ritual, which are arguably central to the practice and role (Newitt 2011, 107): "I've [made] a collection of prayers in different faith traditions ... if prayer would be something a person of a variety of faiths would be interested in" (Annalise, chaplain, Vancouver).

The transition from religious-specific pastoral care has varied in Canada. In some settings, the alternative to pastoral care has been generic spiritual care; elsewhere it has been faith-specific chaplaincy; and there is also a hybrid of the two models in some hospitals. As the Canadian populace has secularized, with lower numbers affiliating with organized religion and attending church, a generic spiritual care model has provided a better fit, reflecting a diverse citizenry, and alignment with the trend toward professionalization of chaplaincy. In the North American CPE model, spiritual care has seen a strategic transformation from a "peripheral service, applicable only to the few 'religious' patients, into an integral element of patient care for all" (Lee 2002, 339). The Vancouver research sites aspired to align with the generic spiritual care model while also providing religion-specific pastoral care at each site. At some sites the model also includes aspects of the UK multi-faith chaplaincy, with volunteers from various faith communities (e.g., Buddhist, Sikh, Hindu, and Jewish) conducting religious services and visitations.

In the United Kingdom, the 1990s was a critical decade for change in the religion-specific chaplaincy or generic spiritual care axis. "The Patient's Charter" (BMJ 1991) prioritized all patients' religious and spiritual needs, regardless of faith tradition. Consequently, healthcare chaplaincy teams have become more multi-faith. Post–Second World War Britain experienced a large migration of South Asian people, with Muslims now 4.8 per cent of the UK population, its second-largest faith group (Gilliat-Ray, Ali, and Pattison 2013, 5), and 12.4 per cent of London's population. This led to the employment of part-time and full-time Muslim chaplains, and the reconfiguring of hospital prayer spaces to meet the needs of various religious traditions (see Gilliat-Ray, Ali, and Pattison 2013).

The concept of multi-faith chaplaincy followed several years' collaboration by various UK chaplaincy bodies, and the emergence of the Multi-Faith Group for Healthcare Chaplaincy. This body has undergone several name changes. Renamed the Network for Pastoral, Spiritual and Religious Care in Health, to reflect recent participation by humanist spiritual caregivers, and a deliberate distancing from the historic Christian terms *chaplain* and *chaplaincy*, the link is restored in its latest name, Healthcare Chaplaincy Forum for Pastoral, Spiritual and Religious Care (as of 2017). The multi-faith ideal was also influenced by the Orchard Report (2000) on London healthcare chaplaincy, which criticized Christian chaplains for acting as brokers for other religious traditions.

One site added *multi-faith* to *chaplaincy* in response to guidance from the Department of Health, which twice mentions multi-faith chaplaincy (DOH 2003, 4–5). *Caring for the Spirit: A Strategy for the Chaplaincy and Spiritual Healthcare Workforce* (South Yorkshire NHS

Workforce Development Confederation 2003), another national initiative, "expected new policy statements in support of multi-faith chaplaincy teams" (paragraph 96). The name change also acknowledged and celebrated the appointment of a part-time imam to the core chaplaincy team. Previously it was predominantly Christian (Church of England, Methodist, and Roman Catholic), with a Jewish lay visitor authorized by the Jewish Visitation Committee.

Another London site serves a high Muslim, Sikh, and Hindu demographic, but their faith representatives are Bank chaplains, paid for regular sessions or occasional call out but not, in this setting, integrated into the core team (in Canada, this type of position would be referred to as casual). Although exclusively Christian, the core chaplaincy team at this site nonetheless has a rich ethnic profile. Its generic model of spiritual care, whereby a Christian chaplain fluent in Indian languages ministered to people of other faith traditions, rather than the appropriate Bank chaplain, appeared to compromise the religion-specific ideal of UK multi-faith chaplaincy, but was probably financially driven as Bank chaplains' visits entail additional cost.

Spiritual Care as Team Responsibility or Specialist Task

The horizontal dimension of the diagram highlights who is responsible for the broad remit of spiritual care. The core question is whether it is predominantly the specialist[4] task of chaplains (VandeCreek and Burton 2001), or a responsibility of the whole healthcare team (Robinson, Kendrick, and Brown 2003, 9; NICE 2004, 99; for the United States, see Balboni, Puchalski, and Peteet 2014, 1587), with professions like nursing playing a distinctive role alongside chaplains (McSherry 2001, 110). De Bono (2012) concludes, on the basis of a review of scholarly literature, that many allied healthcare disciplines are claiming or reclaiming that their scope of practice can address spiritual care issues without chaplains being integrated members on the clinical team. The recent white paper on spiritual care in North America makes a case for a generalist-specialist model parallel to the medical model in which spiritual care generalists (physicians, nurses, social workers) are responsible for assessing spiritual needs and referring to the chaplaincy team when in-depth spiritual care is appropriate (Hall, Hughes, and Handzo 2016).

This axis thus raises questions of training for chaplains and others engaged in spiritual care, like nurses or other healthcare professionals, including what model or models of care should training adopt and equip them for. "Somebody wants to pray and ... if that's not in your understanding, we'll educate you" (Paul, chaplain, London). This question connects with wider debates about the influences of models of healthcare – medical (Norwood 2006), bio-psycho-social (Balboni, Puchalski, and Peteet 2014, 1589), or in which spirituality is incorporated (Raffay, Wood, and Todd 2016). As Annalise noted, "If the problem ... leans more to a medical model, that's not helping ... the psychosocial, emotional, spiritual stuff." The interaction of different models in the context of spiritual care inevitably influences chaplains' approach to prayer with patients; for example, where their prayer offers hope, even when the medical prognosis suggests otherwise, their language negotiates the ambivalence. Margaret, a London chaplain, explained: "I pray for healing, but I never pray for recovery. I don't think *recovery* is a very good word to use."

Negotiation along this axis includes the chaplain's membership on the multidisciplinary team. In one Vancouver unit, "spiritual health has ... an equal spot, a legitimate spot" (Taryn). The fuller integration of the spiritual care team into multidisciplinary teams at Vancouver sites (as illustrated in our chapter 4 comparisons) contrasts with chaplaincy's involvement at our London sites typically confined to particular clinical specialties via the weekly multidisciplinary team meetings concerned with, for example, palliative care, HIV patients, and the social needs of families on a neonatal unit. With fewer chaplains, the London chaplaincy teams had to prioritize their deployment and, while less obvious, this is also true of the Vancouver teams. Our research settings have longstanding examples of inter-professional cooperation, and growing commitment to a transpersonal model integrating physical, psychosocial, and spiritual dimensions of care. London chaplain Paul believed, "There is now greater awareness by many staff that what is agitating the person isn't physical care ... and they want to say prayers."

An inadvertent effect of a strong chaplaincy representation at our Vancouver sites (see chapter 4) was that spiritual care was viewed as a specialist task, to be left to the designated spiritual care team. During interviews, healthcare professionals spoke about their referrals to the spiritual care team, but few understood spiritual care as their own responsibility beyond being supportive to patients and families, and ensuring chaplains were called. In the following excerpt, Shanice (healthcare professional, Vancouver) imagined sending a referral to chaplaincy, rather than responding directly to a patient's request:

> RESEARCHER: So if a patient or a family member requests prayer or a similar spiritual practice on your floor, what happens? What happens at night?
> SHANICE: I think people would make a referral. Unless they directly say to me, "Can you pray for me?" Then you would get them in touch with or if they need to speak to a priest you just get them in touch with Spiritual Care, Pastoral Care team.

As an exception, another healthcare professional said she prayed with all her patients, but overall, the team-specialist axis saw a heavy preference toward the specialist end of the continuum in Vancouver.

The axis of spiritual care as team responsibility or specialist task was receiving some attention at our London sites. One site emphasized its multidisciplinary delivery by organizing a conference for healthcare professionals on their responsibility for spiritual care. A similar conference held at another London site showcased the chaplains' specialist role, but also emphasized healthcare professionals' responsibility by issuing them with a Staff Resource outlining spiritual needs across a wide range of religions and belief. Despite these educational initiatives, as with the healthcare professionals at Vancouver sites, those in London saw their role primarily as that of making referrals.

Professionalism or Advocacy

The third dimension, represented by the diagonal axis, engages with chaplaincy identity. It concerns the balance between a chaplain being a health professional akin to, and identifying with, other professions in healthcare; and what distinguishes chaplains from other healthcare professionals, such as identifying with patients as human beings and being their advocate in the specialist world of medicine. Here Curtis stressed the former: "It's not that I have time [for patients].... It's more that I have skill." Also emphasizing professionalism, Paul commented, "Faith and belief ... come into the whole spectrum of need but ... have to be professional. It's not just a matter of walking around the hospital with a holy halo saying prayers." Contrastingly, Wendy, a London chaplain, explained, "You can be an intermediary [between patient and doctor]." In the definition of *chaplaincy* cited above, there are questions about chaplains described as "nominated individuals authorized for this task in secular situations" (Swift, Cobb, and Todd 2015, 2). This phrase encapsulates possible debates about faith community nomination and authorization, within those communities and the healthcare organization where the person works. It raises questions about authority and the chaplain's professional identity as healthcare and/or faith-based practitioner.

The professionalism-advocacy axis takes a particular form at the Vancouver sites in spiritual care volunteers. To demonstrate that spiritual care is integral to healthcare services, professionalism has been emphasized, especially in British Columbia, where, in 2009, Fraser Health Authority (responsible for all healthcare services in a region of Metro Vancouver) eliminated twelve of its fourteen chaplains in a cost-cutting measure. It defended the move by asserting that the so-called non-core service would be provided by social workers and volunteers from faith communities (Todd 2010). This landmark decision demonstrated the vulnerability of spiritual care and the variance across the province in how it was resourced and regulated. In response to considerable lobbying from faith communities and activist chaplains, the minister of health appointed a working group to develop a provincial spiritual health framework. The subsequent Spiritual Health Council and Framework clearly communicates that the majority of spiritual care is provided by professionals, with trained faith-specific volunteers providing religious care and addressing spiritual needs "solely within the context of a specific religion or denomination" (Ministry of Health 2012). Professionalism is emphasized through CPE courses completed by most of our Vancouver chaplaincy participants, and also offered at some of our research sites in Vancouver. CPE education includes foundational knowledge about spiritual care competencies and the CASC Code of Ethics for Spiritual Care Professionals.

In the United Kingdom, the multi-faith ideal coincided with the professionalization of the chaplaincy role. The *Caring for the Spirit* (South Yorkshire NHS Workforce Development Confederation 2003) initiative expected chaplains to demonstrate their evidence base through a minimum data set of their spiritual care, and by being research aware and research active like their multidisciplinary team colleagues. A chaplaincy career structure was proposed (but not progressed) similar to doctors; a commissioned paper (Folland 2006) encouraged chaplaincies to review and update their working models; and an influential review of chaplaincy research was published (Mowat 2008). Several of our chaplaincy participants contributed to the chaplaincy research agenda by publishing their MA dissertations, and this research interest led to collaborative research with other healthcare professionals, as envisaged by *Caring for the Spirit*.

Most UK chaplaincy post advertisements assume voluntary professional registration with the UK Board of Healthcare Chaplaincy (UKBHC), which oversees professional development and has pioneered appropriate disciplinary structures. In August 2017, following several years' rigorous process, UKBHC's register was accredited by the Professions Standards Authority (UKBHC 2020). Although CPE is not a requirement for spiritual caregivers in English hospitals, regular reflective practice and training is encouraged.

THE LIMINALITY OF PRAYER AND CHAPLAINCY

What emerges from the history of chaplaincy, from our study, and the diagram that informs this chapter, is the multiple social and often marginal locations that chaplains occupy. As chaplaincy studies scholars Chris Swift, Mark Cobb, and Andrew Todd (2015, 164) observe, "Healthcare chaplains effectively occupy marginal positions in multiple worlds, ranging from the community of healthcare professionals, to secular management structures and religious bodies." Occupying multiple locations necessitates a range of boundary work for spiritual caregivers, as they move between social domains, negotiating and transgressing the boundaries between them (see further Todd 2015). As anthropologist Frances Norwood (2006) suggests, these marginal locations may be structural, as the result of inequalities of power and hierarchy (principally the biomedical model), or ideological, arising from inequalities of knowledge and practice.

That chaplaincy care involves "intentional recognition and articulation of the sacred" (Swift, Cobb, and Todd 2015, 2) encapsulates a distinctively liminal aspect of the spiritual care role, "pointing out the existence of an alternative reality, embodying and being a threshold between the two" (Threlfall-Holmes and Newitt 2011b, xv). This quotation suggests that prayer, which signifies that alternative reality, is also central to the chaplain's role. This contributes to the idea that chaplains are fringe figures, even though our data show prayer's ubiquity in the modern hospital. Chaplains often recognized their own liminality; for example, Annalise described this reality, which she found most discomforting: "I've got five minutes before the doctor's coming and, 'Hi, can I pray for you?'" The final section of this chapter offers a systematic exploration of such liminality, not least in relation to prayer.

As signalling their crossing and re-crossing of social thresholds, the term *liminal* seems appropriate to describe chaplains' identity. However, this usage does not altogether conform to received anthropological understandings of liminality and, moreover, is under-examined in the chaplaincy literature (see Threlfall-Holmes and Newitt 2011a, xiv–xvii). Anthropologist Victor Turner (1974) locates the experience of liminality in relation to rites of passage (drawing on earlier work by van Gennep 1960). At the heart of the rite, and the liminal experience, is a crisis of identity and social reorientation, involving the crossing of a social threshold. Rites enable the stripping of the initiate's old identity; a period of separation from the main body of society (perhaps with other initiates); the liminal experience of intense togetherness within the separated group, which Turner (1974, 82–3) terms *communitas*; re-entry into mainstream society; and the initiate's reintegration within the normal order or process of society, or *societas* (193), with their new social identity established.

This kind of anthropological analysis assists the identification of one kind of liminal work done by chaplains, which is to accompany patients, carers, and families through some of the rites of passage, or related experiences, that recipients of healthcare may undergo. The chaplain facilitates actual rites, within the liminal space of hospitals, "their strangeness as theological prospect" (Dykstra 1990, as quoted in Coble 2015, 9) associated with the beginning and end of life. Chaplains also nurture the transitional experiences of patients; for example, as they grapple with the identity of being a cancer patient, or with the life-changing effects of surgery. According to Taryn, "Often the staff will call because they don't know what to do." But a Turner-type analysis, as will be seen, does not altogether account for the multiple liminal experiences undergone by chaplains themselves, that reshape their own identity (rather than that of a patient).

A complementary perspective on rites of passage, which offers insight here, is that of philosopher Pierre Bourdieu (1991). Directing attention away from the chronology of rites of passage – the individual's experience of "before and after" – he highlights the boundary work being done. In particular, Bourdieu stresses the importance for the initiates of their inclusion in the group of all who have undergone this rite, or indeed will undergo it. For example, doctors and other healthcare professionals become members of their professional group through the transitional rite of professional examination and qualification.

What is striking about chaplains' own liminal experience centres on this question of the boundary work associated with group membership, and particularly how it is negotiated.[5] This is seen, for example, in research data associated with chaplains' engagement with multidisciplinary teams. Although not universal, some spiritual care providers experienced inclusion in the multidisciplinary team, as in an extract about what took place at a palliative care multidisciplinary team meeting: "And that's where for me, as a chaplain, the prayers I've offered or the spiritual life I've shared with patients, is shared with the doctors, and the doctors share their learning with the chaplains. And it's an amazing mix in that place. And they're amazing doctors. I mean they really listen to Spiritual Care.... And it was chaplaincy that offered the first voice. The first patient experience was the chaplain" (Martin, chaplain, London). Here the chaplain clearly crossed the boundary of the multidisciplinary team. In the context of the palliative care multidisciplinary team meeting, the chaplain combined his chaplaincy identity with that of team member (as other members combine the latter with their own distinct professional identity). Further, he may lead discussion on particular patients, as in this case where chaplaincy "offered the first voice," having had the first patient contact. Niall, a Vancouver chaplain, experienced similar integration: "I didn't have to earn the right to be at the table. I was actually welcomed and … treated with great warmth when I came here."

However, membership on multidisciplinary teams was not necessarily straightforward in our Vancouver and London research sites. For example, at one site, the chaplains had always accessed and written in patients' paper notes, but their application to access and write in the electronic patient record was declined by the site's information guardian, despite the endorsement of a consultant to the palliative care team. Without access to the electronic record, membership on the multidisciplinary team becomes tenuous. Wendy gave another example of negotiated team membership: "We can have input in [the palliative care multidisciplinary team] and are often asked, 'Are you involved with this patient who has been dying?' We're involved with most people, but some decide not to have chaplaincy involvement, which is fine as well. That's where I gave feedback about the medication a patient had requested." This excerpt suggests three things. One: the chaplain's membership on the team meeting was not taken for granted, as it would usually be for a doctor or nurse. Two: the nature of the chaplain's contribution (concerning the feelings of the patient) was also not taken for granted, but needed continuing negotiation. Three: the chaplain's role in this case was linked to advocacy, where she spoke up on behalf of the patient. A comment by Stanley, an administrator at a London site, presumably reflects chaplains' customary membership on multidisciplinary teams there: "I have no objection if a patient says, 'I absolutely want my spiritual adviser to be at my multidisciplinary team meeting. They're absolutely part of my process of care and getting better.' Fine, have him there. But don't just have him there, whatever you are." Yet even in the research sites where chaplains are assigned to clinical teams and the chaplain-patient ratio is higher – a factor that can facilitate their integration – Curtis said, "People trained to look for spiritual distress and strength are in such small numbers in the system that it's a bit like the voice crying in the wilderness."

These data strongly suggest two further and related things about the liminal identity of the chaplain. First, the transition, or crossing the threshold, into group membership is not a once and for all event, associated with professional qualification. Rather, it recurs and needs to be renegotiated, depending on whether the chaplain has relevant experience to share about particular patients. Second, even having crossed the threshold of the team meeting, the chaplain retains a level of marginality. The liminal experience of the chaplain, in relation to joining a multidisciplinary team, may well recur repeatedly (requiring continued social work) and be partial or incomplete. The liminal identity of the chaplain appears semi-permanent, at least within healthcare. Wendy even conceded that, from the biomedical perspective, "they can actually do without me."

Pursuing the question of group membership and professional identity further, if clinicians function within the multidisciplinary team on the basis of their professional healthcare qualification, chaplains do not necessarily participate on the basis of their professional qualification in religious or spiritual care. The threshold of group membership is not a high or demanding one for the clinician, because the liminal transition into a particular team is an extension of the much more demanding prior transition into the clinical domain (through examination and qualification). For the chaplain, however, the threshold of the team is significantly higher and does not necessarily follow from previous transitions into membership of the faith professional's group, or even the chaplaincy profession. Further, the transition is enabled, and the chaplain's participation is permitted by the group, on the basis of utility. To borrow and adapt a phrase from the world of conversation analysis (e.g., Schegloff 2007), the chaplain's contribution must be seen to have "procedural consequentiality" – to be immediately relevant to the discussion of a particular patient. Taryn noted, "Depending on who is leading the team, the space they give to spiritual health differs tremendously. Very rarely in some environments do we assess [spiritual needs] in rounds, unless I speak up and say, 'I've been following this patient.' However, even then, depending on who the staff is." So group membership is contingent and temporary, and that is why the transition into the group must be repeated over time.

Even when accepted into contingent membership of the multidisciplinary team, the chaplain's faith/belief status could continue to transgress the group's norms. Paul described a multidisciplinary Schwartz round[3] that discussed "how ... faith interfered at times with treatment," including a surgeon who said, "You won't be praying over this body" to someone (presumably not a chaplain) who refused to accept that the patient had died. Yet Paul too maintained boundaries, telling unauthorized faith visitors, "You won't be praying at all until you get permission." The ambiguous status of chaplains goes hand-in-hand with recurring and incomplete liminal transitions into groups within the domain of professional healthcare. This is demanding on chaplains. The chaplain never quite achieves full integration into the *societas* (the social structure and process) of public healthcare. Even at the Vancouver research sites where the chaplaincy department was comparatively well resourced and generally valued by administrators, staff, and patients, chaplains retained a liminal presence in that they also spoke about the importance of developing relationships with staff in order to be known, and the need to continually show evidence for the legitimacy of their work. "Administrators are pushing that we have evidence-based [practice]. I just want to do my job. But I understand it. How do you explain to a medical director the value of these things in language that they understand? Like, does it [chaplaincy] cut down on hospital stay dollars?" (Annalise). In many ways chaplains walk "between the worlds of religion and medicine, pastor and clinician, and religious organizations and medical centres" (Cadge 2012, 29).

Perhaps chaplains depend on the recurring liminal quality of their engagement with healthcare in order to provide effective spiritual care, especially in relation to prayer. There is significant evidence from our study of the adaptation or integration of prayer as it is introduced into the healthcare context, particularly generic spiritual care when it is broadened and made as inclusive as possible. Our Vancouver fieldwork revealed a remarkable variety of religious and spiritual practices related to prayer that suggest transgressive work by chaplains who move between sacred and secular, transcendent and immanent. Two social developments in particular have created openness within healthcare services to such practices. First, in what religious scholar Carlos Colorado (2017) refers to as "indigenizing secularism," land acknowledgments and welcome blessings are commonly offered at public gatherings in Canada, as historic gestures of reconciliation that bring sacred language (e.g., thankfulness to the Creator) and spiritual practices (e.g., drumming, singing) into public spaces. Second, many citizens look to traditional (e.g., Chinese medicine, ayurvedic treatments) and complementary healing practices (e.g., reiki, massage) in conjunction with biomedicine, influenced by immigrant communities and New Age spiritualities. "Very few people are pure anything" (Curtis).

At the same time, resistance to prayer could be anticipated; as Jane, a Vancouver chaplain, said of an instance of offering prayer, "I was forcing myself." Yet equally, the performance of prayer is, according to some chaplains, expected: "It's part of the job: you show up and perform" (Mila, chaplain, Vancouver). Like the chaplain's identity, therefore, offering prayer had to be negotiated, but it also retained its otherness and continued to be transgressive. Theologian and chaplain Richard Coble (2015, 11) notes that "as strangers yet intimates, chaplains are locked in a perpetual state of not belonging. Liminality, the in-between, becomes a part of our identity, an identity always escaping us. The breakage we find in the midst of the intimate encounter is a part of ... who we are." Sociologist Masoud Kianpour (2013, 75) warns chaplains that these encounters risk stress and burnout, and yet for patients and caregivers this "human connection" is the prerequisite of effective spiritual care (Selman et al. 2018, 225).

While the expression of prayer within healthcare offered benefits to patients, it was precisely the otherness of prayer that spoke to, touched, or enabled patients in their experience of the liminality of undergoing healthcare. This key aspect of the chaplain being present with a patient in that liminal place is evident from the following extract, which also illustrates the broadening of prayer within the healthcare context: "If I go for a walk with a patient into the park, just sitting with the patient on the bench and being in the midst of nature, you know, flowers or trees. That could be considered a form of prayer, being in communion with God and part of God's creation. [*Hesitates.*] I don't think I widen the scope of prayer too much on that because you could almost say prayer is everything. So for me I think it's primarily a form of communion using some form of language or communication tool, speaking, listening" (Niall, chaplain, Vancouver). Particularly significant here is the word "communion," used first within a traditional theological register (albeit in a non-ecclesial setting), and then again within a wider, more inclusive register. It signals, in keeping with other data, the deep relationality of praying with a patient (akin to the practitioner's relationship with God), however inclusive the form.

The communion of prayer is therefore close to the *communitas*, the intense and unstructured relationality, discovered by those undergoing a rite of passage, especially the phase between separation from mainstream society and reintegration within it (van Gennep 1960). Indeed, *communion* is used by Turner (1974, 82) as a cognate of *communitas*. This would confirm that this kind prayer, while located within the domain of healthcare, remains Other to that setting and as such supports and enables the liminal experience of the patient. It further suggests that the chaplain's ability to accompany the patient, to offer prayer, is enabled by the fact that chaplains too have some location within the domain, but also remain Other to it, in the recurring liminality of their work and social identity.

National history and policy affect the relative position of our research sites on the three axes of spiritual care outlined in this chapter, though in both Canada and the United Kingdom chaplaincy has become increasingly generic and professionalized. Our study nevertheless suggests that chaplains constantly renegotiate their membership on multidisciplinary teams, a liminal experience related to their prayerful connection with those in their care. This liminality contributes to the transgressive nature of prayer, where it may be deemed not to belong in the biomedical world. Chaplains also adjust their approaches to care, depending on clinical contexts and populations cared for – the theme we turn to in the next chapter.

Prayer amongst the Many:
Clinical Settings and Populations

Sheryl Reimer-Kirkham, Rachel Brown, and Christina Beardsley

This chapter explores those times and places when prayer is integrated into clinical care. In our project, prayer showed up most commonly in times of crisis or at the end of life, but also in other times and places such as long-term care and mental health settings, and with a variety of people, including patients and staff who may be on the margins of society on account of their social positioning or circumstances. Illness can create situational vulnerability for anyone and can also exacerbate conditions of structural vulnerability[1] for those who are already disadvantaged in some way. In the words of Wendy, a chaplain in London, "In a hospital, everyone is equal to a point. Because all are vulnerable, the most wealthy person becomes quite vulnerable. They lose their dignity, they can't look after themselves, they have to put up with all sorts of indignity. But I think poor people are most vulnerable. My empathy goes towards the street person and the more vulnerable or poverty-stricken person. If we have a street person who dies and there is no next of kin, I like to follow through. There may be only the undertaker and myself." In the face of such vulnerability, the task of healthcare professionals and chaplains is, in the widely referenced aspiration of chaplaincy studies scholar Lawrence Holst, "to help the patient retain their personhood apart from the devastation of their illness" (1973, 35).

It is beyond the scope of this chapter to enter into philosophic or theological debates about personhood[2] and holism.[3] Rather we proceed from the stance that each individual is distinct and integrated (i.e., with interdependence between mind, body and spirit), with the capacity to engage with others. The human spirit, vital to personhood, is described by theologian John Swinton (2001, 14) as "the essential life-force that undergirds, motivates and vitalizes human existence." Maryanne, a Vancouver administrator, articulated the relevance of personhood this way: "To me it's looking after the spirit of the person. Where I see that it gets lost a lot of times in healthcare is that we as providers get caught up in the tasks and the doing, so we forget that we're looking after the whole person." Personhood is always evolving in a combination of selfhood (what theologian Alistair McFadyen [1990] refers to as a "deep self"), interpersonal interactions, and macro-level social influences, what feminist religious studies scholar Chris Klassen refers to as "the permeability of all living existence" (2016, 184). Too often the structural nature of suffering and crisis are overlooked (see Introduction), and this relates to prayer as well. The emphases on divine intervention, spirit, and personhood that typically accompany prayer can inadvertently obfuscate social suffering and the structural vulnerabilities that result in negative health outcomes.

In the remainder of this chapter, we explore how prayer showed up "amongst the many." Following from chapter 1, we apply an analytic framework – presenting the context, forms, and intentions of prayer – to structure our discussion of prayer in five clinical settings: critical care, palliative care, long-term care, mental health, and street clinics. Our reference to "the many," however, extends beyond these specialties to a social reading of prayer's imbrications with structural vulnerabilities. In so doing, we gain insights into the contextual nature of prayer, how prayer offered a sense of presence in these varying clinical and social contexts, and the transgressive nature of prayer.

CRITICAL CARE: PRESENCE IN CRISIS

I lost a limb. Or my baby died. These are messy imperfect places. I feel there is a lot of invitation for prayer.

Taryn, chaplain, Vancouver

Loss and crisis are common to critical care units in hospitals and can bring into focus the more existential elements of life (Coble 2018). Critical care is the specialized care of patients who face a life-threatening condition that involves the immanent failure of vital system organs, typically delivered in an intensive care unit (ICU), Emergency Department (ED), or other complex care units. The invasive and highly technical nature of the environment, difficulty in communicating with an unconscious patient, and dehumanizing aspects of care were noted by our participants as both obscuring spiritual dimensions of caregiving and bringing them to the fore as matters of ultimate concern in the face of life and death. In the words of Stanley, an administrator, "You're up against heady mixtures of birth and death, aren't you? And things like termination of pregnancy and fertility, these are at the heart of being human." Crisis is a common denominator of critical care in that these acute episodes of illness often come unexpectedly, whether as trauma or the exacerbation of disease. Chaplains were often called to support patients and families in crisis, such as during a Code (resuscitation by a highly trained team responding to patients who have suffered cardiac or respiratory failure). They described entering "spaces where people are caught, numb, in shock." Taryn explained, "There's nothing else to do but be in this space of pain and confusion. Once we're in that space and there is a sense of acknowledgment that we're in this space together, that's when I may ask the question of prayer."

In some cases, families asked for or expected prayer in times of crisis, while in other cases it was the chaplain who offered prayer, as indicated in the foregoing quote. In these crises, forms of prayer aligned with and countered what one might expect. Prayer typically occurred at bedsides or in waiting rooms, rather than in designated sacred spaces (such as a chapel). Priests spoke of bringing Holy Communion and Anointing of the Sick to the bedside of critically ill patients. Most prominent in the data were informal prayers offered in the moment. As a chaplain, Frances (Vancouver), put it, "There's no formal prescription for how it should go. It's to allow the patients or families to be guiding it." Several chaplains spoke about their role in accompanying families while viewing their loved one in the morgue, who might request prayer to "release the spirit," or that the loved one be "received into the arms of God." An excerpt from Taryn's research diary reveals much about prayer in times of crisis:

> I received a request at 2 a.m. to see a family whose mother had
> just passed away. When I arrived, the mother was lying peacefully
> in her bed, covered with a thick, leopard-print blanket, eyes
> closed, with about eight family members around the room. This
> was a First Nations family whose mother identified as Christian,

but the family was unsure of what denomination, whether Catholic or Protestant. The relatives in the room didn't practise Christianity and one was an ardent Atheist. They asked for "prayers" but didn't know how to describe what they meant by prayer. I had some concerns because I wasn't sure of how my own evangelical Christian tradition and "style" of prayer would bump into their ideas and request. I gained permission to use the language of "God" because their mom referred to "God," and I was also granted freedom to pray as I would naturally. After sharing memories of the patient and asking for specific suggestions to pray about from the family, I prayed a non-formal prayer and incorporated the family's wishes that the patient would be "free" and that the sister would be able to cope with the news.

In crisis moments, the acuity, immediacy, and unexpectedness of the situation often preclude pre-existing relationships with the patient/family. As a result, Taryn carefully followed the family's lead in ascertaining who the prayer would be addressed to and the nature of the concerns to be expressed in the prayer. She wrote with self-awareness about the risk of imposing her own style, which she described as "evangelical." This case illustrates navigating diversity in prayer, where those involved held various religious identities. Together and in the moment, they found a common vocabulary for prayer. Numerous stories in our study evidenced situations in which there was no concordance between the religious affiliations of those praying, and yet deep connection and meaning was achieved (see chapter 7).

For most participants, the intentions of prayer in critical care contexts were not primarily religious (i.e., to do with deity or God or formal religious practices) but were more often intended to support the expression of ultimate concerns, to offer care in the face of suffering, and to create an atmosphere of peace or healing. Frances told the story of a distraught daughter whose mother had just arrived in Emergency: "I ask, 'Is there any way we could help you?' She says, 'I would like to pray, but I don't know how, because this is too critical, it's too overwhelming, I can't think.' Finding out she is Catholic, I ask, 'Would you like a rosary?' She looks in her bag and can't find one and she's even more panicky. I bring her one, place it in her hand.... I see her shoulders go down and she finds her space. It helped her to settle, cope, breathe." Here the chaplain was closely tuned to how prayer, with the familiarity and materiality of the rosary, could provide care for an anxious family member, such that prayer could create a sense of "peace, calmness, and not let the confusion of the critically acute situation take over." Prayer could transgress the pre-eminence of bio-medical interventions and the common mechanical view of life and death, where life is evaluated by biometric readings of body function.

PALLIATIVE CARE: PRESENCE AS ACCOMPANYING

There's an expectation of prayer in the traditional sense in end-of-life care settings, whether prior to or after death.

Ronald, chaplain, Vancouver

Palliative care patients and their families are dealing with incurable, life-threatening illness. The medical focus is on improving "quality of life ... through the prevention and relief of suffering by means of early identification and impeccable assessment and treatment of pain and other problems, physical, psychosocial and spiritual" (World Health Organization n.d.). Pioneered in cancer settings, palliative care has been extended to a range of non-malignant conditions, including progressive neurological disease, and to well before the terminal or end-of-life stage. Influenced by a number of hospice pioneers (see Fitchett and Nolan 2015, 195), spirituality is usually well-integrated in this area of medicine. The holistic model developed by nurse and physician Cicely Saunders (n.d.), with its sensitivity to the internal or spiritual pain that can accompany dying (for both patients and their loved ones) has been especially influential.

Some of our research sites had dedicated palliative care teams. Chaplains were members of these multidisciplinary teams, and spiritual care was prioritized according to national guidance or policy. One chaplain who had an office on the Palliative Care Unit felt "pretty tight" with that team, contributing to its decisions, but less involved in the Emergency Department, "where there's no space for me.... It's the presence that makes the difference and people know what you really do." Noting that spirituality is discussed as a component of care at weekly team meetings, Ezra (chaplain, London) observed, "But that is relatively unique to palliative care, end-of-life care ... compared to other clinical areas, for pretty obvious reasons." The main reason is the imminence of death. Zara, a London healthcare professional accustomed to assessing spiritual needs, agreed that "the way we incorporate it [prayer] is often at the end of life.... [T]hat's when we start to ask them." Emma, another healthcare professional in London, said, "Care should be holistic. It shouldn't just be physical." Strong links between the hospitals' palliative care teams and local hospices, where some members were also employed, enabled that.

Paul, a chaplain also working at a London hospice, regarded the hospice as "in some ways more conducive to pray[er]." This related partly to facilities, "individual rooms and ... small meeting rooms," but also to ethos. "The staff are aware that dying is very much part of the daily occurrence and ... very supportive and welcoming to chaplaincy." Creating appropriate spaces and atmosphere meant that Vancouver's Palliative Care Unit "has a very different feel. It's intentionally supposed to feel different" (Mila, chaplain). Two London sites have individual designated side-rooms, called Butterfly Rooms (presumably because the butterfly's life is short) on some wards to care for people at the end of life. Hannah, a chaplain who attended someone dying in one of these rooms, declared, "I think that's one of the most wonderful things ever, is those Butterfly Rooms."

Formal prayers, including rites and ceremonies, appeared prominently in the palliative care data, as reflected in Ronald's quote at the beginning of this section. Catholic and other chaplains engaged in this task. Because Pagans are more likely to call on a friend for informal prayer than on her services, Hannah assumed that in hospital "what is most comforting and sought after is ceremony rather than prayer," but this ritual, like more conventionally religious ones, was also about "meditative attunement ... a place of stillness and centredness and from that, personal comfort." These formal prayers were often in conjunction with a listening presence, reflecting the accompanying typical to spiritual care in this setting. Paul, although himself a chaplain, called the priest if sacramental care was required, when "requested to pray with people, especially when people have died," but if "they just want some comfort ... in many cases, I do all the things." Simon, a London chaplain, offered the Lord's Prayer, though the need often turned out to be listening. "Usually we talk, and I suppose that's a kind of prayer, because they tell me how they're feeling." Ronald gave his perspective: "The typical spiritual care: [the] analogy of walking alongside and when you pray with somebody you are actually not submitting a request to the gods but finding a way to lift up the current situation. Often the form is 'lament' and involves to 'pray with.'

Which is different than 'pray for.'" One of our London chaplains described his shift from praying set prayers from a book to "what I interact with" – in this example, someone diagnosed with motor neurone disease. In language that echoed the face-to-face relational philosophy of Emmanuel Lévinas (see Ford 1999), he said that spirituality "will be defined by the two people interacting. It has a face maybe, but that face is with the person who is interacting with me." Cicely Saunders (n.d.) believed that the spiritual accompanier is "not there to take away or to explain or even understand" but simply "sharing the pain" (Kirkpatrick 1988) that contains its own resolution. Martin, a chaplain in London, described this interaction when people "don't want to be on their own but don't necessarily want to talk. Their brain is asking all the questions they want to ask, and sometimes that whole dynamic is facilitated by the chaplain being at the bed next to them, without breaking the atmosphere. So silence can be very much of a prayerful interaction with another person. If I'm respectful of that silence, then whole-flourishing is going to happen." As Ronald noted, "Silence is a form of prayer," and "sometimes it's not helpful praying when you have spiritual distress." When a dying friend, "a complete Atheist," declined the offer of prayer, Martin invited the friend to hold his hand, and the invitation was accepted. "So I've held hands with somebody for an hour, saying nothing" (see chapter 8).

These encounters of prayer, with their emphasis on the dying person's initiative, illustrated the intention to create that "safe space at the end-of-life for considering ... ultimate questions," a "space in which personhood is protected and dignified as the inevitable losses unfold," quoting nurse researcher Barbara Pesut (2015, 272). This painstakingly attentive interpersonal task resembled Alistair McFadyen's (1990) dialogic account of personhood, which assumes intersubjective communication, mutual understanding, and passive moments, including silence.

LONG-TERM CARE: PRESENCE AS RE-MEMBERING

Four or five times a day, I pass a lovely Hindu gentleman in the hallway, he raises his hand to me, and he bows. I never miss the opportunity to bow towards him and offer him *namaste*. We have done this countless times. Somehow I enter into this sacred space with him. His face is transformed. He has severe dementia, but he'll never forget how to give the bow sign. To me that's an exchange of prayer and blessing. *Namaste* is a blessing of peace. I receive so much from him, and I am giving something to him. It's a sacred moment of prayer.

                                                    Tulio, chaplain, Vancouver

Long-term care[4] for older adults brought into focus how expressions of prayer reminded staff, families, and the residents themselves of the personhood of the older (often frail) person. Although they aspired to provide a home-like setting, care homes had an institutional feel, which could mitigate person-centredness. Many residents suffered from dementia, an overall term for a set of symptoms involving degeneration of cognitive function (e.g., memory loss, executive functions, loss of language abilities, and mood and behavioural disorders) (Alzheimer Society of Canada 2018). Dementia can mean older adults are less communicative about spirituality but, according to psychologists Océane Agli, Nathalie Bailly, and Claude Ferrand's (2015) systematic review of fifty-one articles, they may also benefit from religion/spirituality on account of related coping strategies, meaning making, and social support.

In our study, dementia created unique opportunities and challenges for the expression of prayer. Referencing older adults, chaplains observed that "this generation" was more familiar with prayer, especially in its formal and institutional forms. Prayer was most often described as theistic within the parameters of specific faith traditions. Residents here were reportedly more likely to ask for or expect prayer, compared to other settings, likely because of their familiarity with prayer and the long-term relationships they often had with chaplains (Reimer-Kirkham et al. 2018). Prayer could thus position an older person into a relational sphere, raising the question of whether those residents who conversely were not interested in participating in prayer might be excluded in some way.

Forms of prayer in long-term care settings were described as more formal and yet social and relational. With these formal expressions of prayer during religious services, the exteriority of prayer was evident – as Tulio said, "Prayer thrives in community." Services were offered in keeping with various faith traditions; one site, for example, had Catholic Mass, Christian hymn singing, Buddhist chanting, Indigenous healing ceremonies, and Sikh, Hindu, and Muslim prayers. Sikh residents were taken on daytrips to the *gurdwara* for prayers and *langar*.[5] However, there were also many situations in which connection was achieved not through matching religious affiliations, but rather through a sense of shared respect or human-ness, as reflected in the above narrative of *namaste*. The relational aspects of prayer were also evident in the stories recounted about staff, many of them diasporic healthcare workers (e.g., Filipina, South Asian), reaching out to chaplains for prayer.

A research diary entry by Megan, a chaplain in Vancouver, captured the forms and intentions of prayer in long-term care settings in the description of a service with older people with advanced dementia, many of whom were unable to speak, walk, or talk.

> I opened and closed the service with short prayers, but I also took the opportunity to pray for residents individually. I went to each person, greeted them, asked if I could pray, knelt beside the wheel-chair, put my hand on a shoulder, and prayed a spontaneous prayer that was based on the passage we had just read. Whatever came to mind.

> Lord, thank you for ———. Please give her the fullness of your life and let your light overcome any darkness in her life. Amen.
> Lord, thank you that you came to be present with us. I pray for ———: help him to know your presence every minute of every day. Amen.
> Lord, thank you that grace and truth come through you. I pray for ——— [who struggles with negative thoughts about herself]. Help her to listen only to the truth of your word and help her to know your abundant grace. Amen.

> I pray more often with this group than with other groups of residents. Perhaps because it is a quiet, more private space, it seems more conducive to individual prayer. Perhaps because it is a small-er group of people, it is more possible to pray for each person. Perhaps I have more compassion for these residents confined not only by the weakness of their bodies but also by the limitations of their minds and the difficulty of communication. But most of all, as a Christian, I believe that praying matters even if people are not rationally comprehending it, even if they are asleep or speak another language or cannot hear, no matter how loud I talk. The Lord is working through prayer, so it feels more effective than other kinds of ministry (talking, listening, singing). (Megan, chap-lain, Vancouver)

Several intentions were evident in this account. We observed the chaplain's concern to affirm the dignity and humanity of each individual, even when cognitive functioning and decision-making had declined. She prayed to comfort and encourage, with phrases such as "help her" or "give him." In this excerpt and in other interviews, chaplains talked about prayer in the context of dementia as a way to reconnect older people to their religious/spiritual identity. Here the work of anthropologist Barbara Myerhoff on remembrance is instructive: "The term 're-membering' calls attention to the re-aggregation of members, the figures who belong to one's life story, one's own prior selves, as well as significant others who are part of the story. Re-membering then, is a purposive, significant unification" (as quoted in De Bono 2012, 226).

MENTAL HEALTH: PRESENCE DURING (DIS)CONNECTION

I'm interested in the difference between people's spiritual experiences and voices, versus a psychotic experience.

Elizabeth, healthcare professional, London

Elizabeth, who described herself as a devout person of faith hid her own spirituality from her colleagues, fearing reprisal, and yet saw spiritual experiences intertwined with mental health for the patients whom she cared for. The clinical specialty of psychiatry has long held an uneasy relationship with spirituality and religion, whereby Sigmund Freud's assessment of religion as a "universal obsessional neurosis" has resulted in continued suspicion and pathologizing of religion. Research suggests that, for psychotic patients, incorporating religious and spiritual themes into their delusions may lead to stronger conviction in delusional beliefs, greater severity of symptoms, lower levels of function, and less compliance with psychiatric treatment (Griffith 2012; Weber and Pargament 2014). The last decades, however, have seen a more balanced approach to religion and spirituality, with evidence of both deleterious and salutary effects on mental health. Researchers have, for example, studied the link between psychological distress and spiritual struggles (Ellison and Lee 2010) and have identified that religion and spirituality can be damaging to mental health by negative religious coping, misunderstanding and miscommunication, and negative beliefs (Weber and

Pargament 2014). As a positive force, religion and spirituality may, for example, support positive coping, be a source of community and support, and foster religious beliefs and practices shown to enhance life satisfaction and morale (Weber and Pargament 2014). Many of our participants were tuned to these dynamics. Elizabeth voiced caution: "In mental health particularly, people are really anti-religion, because they think the church is unhealthy for people's mental health." Reflecting the relevance of spirituality to mental health and a different social and organizational context, Taryn noted that "the place I get asked to pray the most is mental health in-patient units." At some in-patient psychiatry units, chaplains were well integrated into multidisciplinary teams, to the extent that psychiatrists prescribed spiritual care visits in some cases. Prescribing prayer as intervention risks the medicalization of prayer on one hand, and on the other suggests the relevance of spiritual support and connection during mental illness.

Forms of prayer varied remarkably in the context of psychiatric care, perhaps more so than in other settings. The chaplains on the in-patient psychiatric unit facilitated various groups, such as discussion groups, and art and music activities. Andreas, a chaplain who integrated contemplative and spiritual practices, explained,

> My work is not just pure prayer or pure meditation. I am creating a healing zone. They want to listen to chanting, they want to say words, they want to read prayers, they want to be quiet, they want to have beads or rosaries, they want to get communion, they want to have the evil-eye in their pocket. They want to do mandalas, they want to write, they want to have a repetitive activity. There are many kinds of prayer. But certainly, what all this does is engage someone's depth, in a bigger, mysterious, unconscious or superconscious connectedness with God. Or maybe not with God but with one another, maybe with the universe.

Notably, very few participants spoke of prayer in the hospital's designated sacred spaces when talking about prayer in relation to mental health. Rather spaces such as a Contemplation Room were where prayer took place on mental health units. Other participants spoke about prayer while walking or sitting in a park with a patient from the mental health unit, as was the case of the chaplain accompanying a patient on a smoke break.

Intentions in the context of mental health and especially the role of the chaplain on multidisciplinary teams involved purposeful movement toward goals of care over time. Taryn told us, "I find it different from other teams, because during rounds the staff will actually ask, 'What are your goals with this patient?' I might say, 'I've worked on meditation, relaxation, or self-compassion.'" Such goals reflect the desire to remind patients of their worth and wholeness, and this meant the chaplain saw them as more than their disease, often visiting "without an agenda" other than affirming their worth as persons. In this way the movement toward prayer was patient-led, contingent upon the trust that had slowly accrued. The intention of prayer could then involve encouragement and strengthening those who might be discouraged, regretful, or struggling with guilt. Niall (chaplain, Vancouver) stated, "Sometimes it's for guidance, sometimes patients are not sure about the way forward, they're confused. Sometimes patients are feeling beaten up by life through ongoing suffering, and so we pray for strength, that there's still life around us, there's still some good things happening. Sometimes it's reminding patients of the promises of God, that he won't leave us or forsake us." Unique to this setting, chaplains needed to take particular care in differentiating between health-promoting and deleterious effects of prayer, being careful not to reinforce delusions or psychosis. Andreas spoke insightfully about such differentiation, noting his role in bearing witness to delusions as part of human experience, while gently, over time, reminding psychotic patients of who they were. He was emphatic about not praying with them during active psychosis, as this carried risk of exacerbating their condition.

STREET CLINICS:
PRESENCE DURING SOCIAL EXCLUSION

I went over to the church next door and told the minister there that we needed to start a prayer therapy workshop together.

Ersi, healthcare professional, London

Street clinics are a form of primary healthcare that seek to provide convenient low-barrier access to healthcare services by reducing the economic and organizational factors that may preclude those who are structurally vulnerable or face social exclusion from receiving the health and social care they require. Street clinics are often situated in neighbourhoods that have higher rates of homelessness, deprivation, or substance use (such as intravenous drug use) and typically operate within a harm-reduction philosophy. Harm-reduction programs aim to meet substance users where they are, rather than imposing a pre-scribed abstinence-based intervention model of care upon them (Marlatt and Witkiewitz 2010).

Two street clinics, though serving different populations and located in different countries, offered an unusual vantage point where prayer showed up. In London the clinic provides care to LGBTQIA popula-tions who may experience difficulty in accessing responsive health and social services. The Vancouver clinic offers supervised injection for intravenous drug users and a range of health and social services with a multidisciplinary team, including spiritual care. A dispropor-tionate percentage of the clientele are Indigenous, as those within Canadian society who are most structurally vulnerable on account of the intergenerational trauma suffered through the cultural assimila-tionist policies of the state- and church-run residential schools of the past century.

Prayer showed up in expected and unexpected ways and forms in the street clinics – sometimes formal, sometimes informal, sometimes clinically bound and sometimes embodied. In Vancouver, where the community has been struggling with how to handle the grief and experience of loss that is present with the opioid crisis,[6] formal prayer services have been an important part of the spiritual care on offer at the clinic. An organization-wide memorial service for the vic-tims, and the clients and staff who knew them, was held at a local park. Smaller-scale services were held at the clinic when someone died. Liam told us, "When somebody passes, we like to put up a little sign or photo of the person with a candle. We will leave it up for a week and maybe make a poster or card where people can sign their name, make some comments. because it's important.... [I]t's another spiritual moment. We need some way to acknowledge that there's been a change or a passing" (healthcare professional, Vancouver). Prayer and related spiritual practices also showed up in the London street clinic where Ersi described the use of mindfulness meditation,[7] especially when a patient is "very anxious." She kept scripts for this practice on her phone for easy access. If she did not have time to lead them through a mindfulness meditation or if she felt that what had happened in their session was "too much ... I will suggest that they go and sit next door in the church for a few minutes just to give themselves some time to process." This perspective is a fascinating one, since the participant discussed prayer as "not part of her role" and yet was ready to lead her patients through mindfulness meditation.

The intentions for prayer in the street clinics were not primarily religious; rather, therapeutic intentions were common, with prayer as a means for connection to the whole self and to others. Ersi explained that she also used prayer therapy to bridge the "interrupted connection" between the body, the mind, and the spirit that is evident in many clients.

> The reason why they end up here is because something about that connection has been interrupted. It can get interrupted by unhelpful means ... by being in the wrong relationships ... because of drugs, because of alcohol, because of fantasies, because of a lot of things. If there is a healthy connection between body and mind, then we assume that will be the way for having healthier sex. Ultimately what they want to achieve is the mind and body to connect in a healthy way where there are no disruptions. Now in my head, that ultimate goal is not different from meditation. My very first homework for the patient will be, "Can you return to your prayers? Can you return to your spiritual practice?"

She described how Muslim men returned to their prayer practices quite easily, but that many non-Muslim men did not have a similar familiarity with prayer. This was the reason for the prayer workshop mentioned in the opening quotation of this section. From that start, Ersi and the minister have facilitated several sessions with encouraging results. She observed that many of the men who participated in the group had been discriminated against for their sexuality within their religious communities, and for their religious identity within the LGBTQIA community: "It's not common to be gay and to also admit to being Christian." She went on to say, "This has been a really supportive network. They realize, 'I'm not alone. I'm not the only gay Christian' ... and that's why we wanted to do it." Ersi was convinced that by finding support in this community, they would eventually support themselves as well.

A similar concern for a whole-person approach to care and social inclusion is evident in the words of Liam: "The medicine and the treatment we provide [referring to medical-grade heroin and hydromorphone] are essential but of minimal importance. The more important aspect is the holistic approach, and that must include spirituality. Unless we can meet someone as an individual, not as a disease, then we're not doing the work we need to do." According to Maryanne, prayer in this context and with this intention in mind was "not necessarily having them connect to God or a higher being, but having them to at least start to connect with the world around them" and "acknowledge themselves as human beings and people of value."

PRAYER AS PRESENCE AND TRANSGRESSION

In this last section we summarize how prayer showed up "amongst the many" in clinical settings. As a first point, regardless of setting, a common thread was the relational and connective aspects of prayer as prerequisite. The motivation for this connection was a profound regard for the personhood of each individual. Prayer was constructed as presence with another, more so than connecting with the divine or a Higher Being, reflected in Ronald's comment of "praying with" rather than "praying for." What varied by setting was the focus or nature of this presence:

> *Critical care – presence in crisis.* Chaplains and healthcare professionals were required to be highly responsive to circumstances, quickly reading relational dynamics in order to ascertain how to be present in a calming, supportive, and humanizing way.
> *Palliative care – presence as accompanying.* Here chaplains and healthcare professionals focused their presence on companioning, listening, and sharing silence. The "deep listening" and "in-depth" encounters that occurred might seem unusual to observers and yet were "normal" for chaplains (Mitchell 2015, 263).
> *Long-term care – presence as re-membering.* The presence of prayer was offered to recall what was meaningful to people with dementia, and in this way to continually affirm them as they had been and still were.
> *Mental health – presence during (dis)connection.* Prayer in this context was carefully offered as a means of bringing wholeness to people disconnected from themselves and others.
> *Street clinic – presence during social exclusion.* Here prayer served as a social presence to counter the social exclusion experienced because of substance use, racialized identity, sexual identity, or other forms of structural vulnerability.

Prayer has been described as a "communicative act" (Collins 2015, 207), typically aimed at communicating with God or a higher being (see chapter 1). In these mobilizations of prayer as presence, the communicative act was also interpersonal with healing intentions. These setting-specific variations carry implications for spiritual care, whether by chaplaincy, healthcare professionals, volunteers, or families, in understanding the specialized nature of each setting, the types of illness experience, and how to adjust one's presence and prayers accordingly. Chaplaincy studies are seeing a trend toward specialization by clinical area or population (see chapter 5; Fitchett and Nolan 2015), and our exploration of "prayer amongst the many" supports such a trend.

As a second point, while the forms of prayer varied, its transgressive nature did not. In each clinical setting, prayer encountered and transgressed biomedical priorities. The reader may well have sensed prayer entering the existential, liminal spaces between living and dying, sanity and insanity, inclusion and exclusion in our descriptions.

Living and dying. Perhaps the most obvious instances of transgression between life and death were when prayer happened immediately before, during, or shortly after death, such as when chaplains prayed with families in a waiting room adjoining the ICU during resuscitation of a loved one, or in the morgue's viewing room. In such situations, prayer was unbounded by time, blurring the lines between life and death. Sociologist Michael Mason (2013, 22) explains: "Prayer takes place in sacred time, conceived as an eternal now. Within the sacred world, clock time is irrelevant.... [T]he time-bound world appears as merely a temporary arrangement."

Sanity and insanity. When prayer is viewed as enchantment, as put forward by sociologist Giuseppe Giordan (2015), the lines between rationality and irrationality are inherently blurred, not unlike experiences of mental illness. Prayer by its very nature involves the world of everyday life intertwined with alternative worlds (Mason 2013, 18). Prayer could offer a grounding presence in the liminal space between sanity and insanity. Anthropologist Tanya Luhrmann (2013, 4) writes, "The central (non-theological) act of prayer is paying attention to internal experience – thoughts, images, and the awareness of one's body – and treating these sensations as important in themselves." This level of deep attention to the internal self, together with an outward turn toward God or other meaningful phenomena or people, was important for prayer as a grounding presence.

Inclusion and exclusion. Prayer was employed to transgress social lines of inclusion and exclusion, as was particularly evident in the settings of long-term care, mental health, and street clinics. Prayer could serve as social bridging capital (Bramadat 2005; Putnam 2000), as seen in the offering of *namaste* with the older Hindu man and in relationships with those struggling with mental health and addictions. For others, as in the cases of the Pagan and Atheist patients, expressions of caring in the face of suffering could take on forms of meditation and prayer when these were person-centred and untethered from religious power, symbols, and meanings. Yet bringing prayer into the vulnerabilities of illness and hospitalization, with prayer's histories and capacities for symbolic violence (Woodhead 2015b, 220), could do great harm and ultimately act as a line of social exclusion rather than inclusion. For the most part, the participants in our study mitigated this harm with the high value they placed on honouring the experiences, values, and beliefs of each individual with whom they interacted.

Our exploration of "prayer amongst the many" portrays the contexts, forms, and intentions of prayer in different settings. Returning to the earlier reference to chaplaincy studies scholar Lawrence Holst's (1973, 35) wise counsel to "help the patient retain their personhood apart from the devastation of their illness," the narratives presented in this chapter demonstrate how prayer can contribute to such ends during times of crisis, loss, disconnection, and exclusion. In the next chapter we look closely at how religious identities are fluid and negotiated during prayer encounters.

Complicating Religious Identities through the Social Relations of Prayer

Rachel Brown, Paul Bramadat, and Sylvia Collins-Mayo

Prayer crosses so much. It crosses people's lives. It crosses faith traditions, religions.

Jane, chaplain, Vancouver

In a book about religion, spirituality, prayer, and identities in health-care settings, readers and writers would hope to operate out of a common understanding of what it means to be a member of this or that religion in this or that setting. Yet immediately our interdisciplinary project runs headlong into the complexities represented by sui generis, lived, and intersectional approaches to religion. When looking at real, lived lives, we see that all three approaches inform and rely on the others to some extent. The puzzle we face in this chapter on identities is what we have in mind when we say that Paresh (a healthcare professional) is a Sikh, or Grace (a patient) is a Christian. We might mean, on the surface, that Paresh calls himself a Sikh and Grace calls herself a Christian and leave the analysis there. Or we could let the individuals decide what or who they are, and how they ought to act. Our task as scholars could just be to reflect on the ways institutional stakeholders respond to these de facto Sikh and Christian claims and expectations. However, our aim in this chapter is to go beyond the surface. We seek to engage with the complexities of religious identities, their intersectional influences, and how they are worked out in the social relations of prayer. Our exploration brings to light the transgressive nature of prayer in blurring lines of identity.

THEORETICAL APPROACHES
TO THE STUDY OF RELIGIOUS IDENTITIES

In the field of religious studies, our focus indicates our interest in the lived religion perspective. This approach to the study of religion is a relatively recent addition to the field (e.g., Hall 1997; Orsi 2003) usually thought to add to, nuance, and complicate the more conventional sui generis perspective (McCutcheon 1997). The latter approach is by far more common and, as that Latin phrase suggests, assumes there is something unique and irreducible about religious ideas and practices. It is linked to the notion that there are a finite number of so-called world religions (usually, Judaism, Christianity, and Islam are framed as the Western or Abrahamic traditions, and Hinduism, Buddhism, Sikhism, and Chinese, and Japanese religions are the Eastern or Asian traditions). In each religion, following the sui generis approach, we would then expect to find coherent ethical, practical, and theological norms – including norms around prayer and praying – rooted in some distinctive set of texts, moral codes, ideas, laws, hierarchies, rituals, and institutions. Many textbooks related to religions of the world, and virtually all political and cultural actors engaged in debates about religion, adopt these assumptions, even while they might acknowledge that each tradition is internally heterogenous to some degree. The general idea, then, from a pure sui generis perspective, is that there is something distinctive about *religious* claims and practices (that is, these are literally, categorically unlike other cultural claims and practices that might be attributed to some other force, such as capitalism, psychology, genetics, and so forth). Moreover, from this perspective most people around the world and throughout history could and can in some meaningful way be said to belong to one of the world religions. Perhaps they are not loyal or devout Sikhs (and so forth), but most people see themselves as members of one of these great and coherent traditions.

Scholars interested in the lived religion perspective might well observe the existence of religious traditions, but they are far more curious about the ways people actually live as Sikhs, Christians, and so on. These scholars agree that the vast majority of individuals would indicate some kind of membership in one of the main world religions (or their smaller offspring, such as Jainism, Unitarianism, and so forth) – therefore bringing some sui generis perspective with them – but wish to find out what that association to a religion means to individuals and what difference it makes to their lives. As noted throughout this project, people seldom live reliably within the bounds of the traditions into which they are born. This is especially true in North America and Western Europe, which are characterized by secularization and in which the social cost of straying outside these boundaries is low. However, even in national contexts in which we might anticipate orthodoxy or homogeneity (rural Italy, for example), individuals negotiate their identities in novel or unpredictable ways. How might we explain the way a devout Italian Catholic, for example, expresses a strong belief in astrology by devoutly listening to Paolo Fox (a popular astrologer in Italy)? The point is simply that while from a certain perspective individuals might be seen, or be said, to belong to one or another of the recognizable world religions (sui generis), upon closer inspection most people belong in their own (lived) ways of religion.

In this project we encountered tensions around sui generis presuppositions about identities being invoked (whether Buddhist, Hindu, Secularist, or Lutheran). This sense of some kind of coherent totality or stable essence of these categories – such as those inferred by the terms Christian or Sikh – is present in the ways people were expected to behave, inside and outside hospital settings. The tension between the sui generis and the lived approaches to religion is in constant conversation and continual flux. Indeed, some institutional settings – legal, educational, and healthcare settings come to mind – incentivize conventional performances of what it might mean to assert that one is part of this or that religious community. The reason is that one's religious identities are typically asserted in these public venues when someone (such as a doctor, patient, lawyer, or plaintiff) is seeking accommodation from the institution itself. Whether they are asking to be allowed to wear a turban, a hijab, or a yarmulke into a courtroom, or to be allocated prayer space or to be served a special diet in a hospital, they are asking, for example, as Jews, Buddhists, or Sikhs (see chapter 2).

Our expectations of norm-following can extend beyond formal requests for special treatment, however. Often we have ideas and ethical stances in mind, too. For example, in the hospital context we might expect that a Buddhist, Hindu, or Sikh who is asked to speak about her view of death will say something about rebirth, or that a Christian patient who is insulted by a hospital roommate will "turn the other cheek." Imagine if Paresh says he believes he has just one life or that he will go to heaven or hell after this life; or if Grace is inclined to strike back at someone who insults her. Well, then we have a dilemma to resolve. Often this dilemma is resolved by assuming that Paresh is simply a "bad" or imperfect Sikh, or that Grace is a hypocrite or just does not understand or care about the emphasis on love in the Bible. In other words, we continue to operate as if having a religious identity means to live in a bounded world (sui generis) whereby lapses or disobediences render claims to this or that identity suspect or at least incomprehensible to other putative members. Throughout this chapter we will see similar examples of situations in which religious individuals do not act according to the scripts we might assume they would follow.

While the dominant sui generis or world religions paradigm most commonly informs understandings of religion and has provided rich and valuable knowledge of religious phenomena, the lived religion approach offers another complex and interesting account of religious phenomena that pays closer attention to the often counterintuitive ways people live their religious lives in the real world. A third approach, drawing on intersectionality, encompasses relatively newer perspectives that focus on how power relations and social structures intersect to affect how religion is lived. For example, intersectionality provides us a lens from which we can observe the ways ordinary people (especially women) experience and construct religious lives for themselves, often against the interests of the elite men who have controlled church and state. Conventional definitions of what it means to be part of a specific religious tradition have typically emanated from the life experiences of elite males within these groups. At best this androcentrism is a consequence of the fact that most socially recognized religious leaders and philosophers responsible for the supposedly key texts, doctrines, and institutions of this or that religion were educated men, and often privileged their personal perspectives (Vincett, Sharma, and Aune 2008).

Debates over immigration, reconciliation with Indigenous people, public space, legal pluralism, and new ways of thinking about our shared heritage often involve claims and assumptions about religion and spirituality. For people trying to understand these contemporary debates, intersectional scholars can help us to pay attention to the ways individuals, groups, and institutions invoke terms such as *religion* (or its specificities, such as Sikhism or Christianity) in ways that are far from transparent. Indeed, because of the sui generis assumptions at work throughout our culture, many people are reticent to treat religious claims and practices in the same ways we treat other sorts of human activity. What this blinds us to are the many ways in which defining a certain space, practice, or role as "religious" can serve as a means of either summarily excluding or naively permitting its ongoing existence.

When the space in question is a publicly funded hospital and the time in question is a "secular" or "post-colonial" period in which many of us are trying to approach subaltern communities and public institutions in sensible ways, we need to think carefully about the ways we come to see particular religious and cultural issues as problems in the first place. For example, many scholars (Bramadat and Kaufert 2013; Garces-Foley 2013; Pesut et al. 2008) have noted that since the 1990s, in the nursing and medical literatures, a concern with "spirituality" has demonstrably come to eclipse "religion." In the last few decades when talking about the ways people experience and talk about suffering and death, the services a hospital might provide, and the ways institutions should identify this particular body of service providers, spirituality has come to be thought of as unproblematic, whereas religion is freighted by its long association (especially in liberal democracies) with colonialism, patriarchy, misogyny, convention, and hierarchy (Bramadat, Coward, and Stajduhar 2013; Garces-Foley 2013). The fact that *spiritual* and *spirituality* are now favoured metaphors or adjectives should not lead us to conclude that they are not also political terms. They are, and their ascendency in the healthcare literature is, just as socially constructed as are our definitions of beauty, justice, and truth. The shift from religion to spirituality in many healthcare settings in Canada and England is political in that it reflects broader shifts in the surrounding society (especially the move toward individualism and neo-liberalism) and comes at a cost to individuals and institutions once, or still, defined as religious. Just as the world religions paradigm reflects a period of the study of religion in which there was fascination with the Other and his or her own essential embeddedness in a given "tradition," and just as the lived religions perspective draws attention to new voices and idiosyncratic negotiations of religious identities, intersectionality provides useful analytic tools to help us think more carefully about the ways religious identities come to be articulated and received in the societies in which we live. Feminist scholar Pnina Werbner (2010) writes that "religious identity is, above all, a discourse of boundaries, relatedness and otherness, on the one hand, and encompassment and inclusiveness on the other – and of the powerful forces that are perceived to challenge, contest and preserve these distinctions and unities" (233).

Here the notion that such identities are discourses is important to remember. They are, in our view, social constructions – ways of talking about the self that are shaped by the societies, languages, and institutions in which these discourses or assertions occur. Whether the self – the "identity" – pre-exists the discursive act that brings it into being is an important question but beyond the scope of this book. What we can say is that in order to understand the way a religious identity might be articulated and might fare in a healthcare setting, it is important to bear in mind (1) the known "facts" about the identity (e.g., what does the sui generis, world religions paradigm tell us about what it means that Paresh is a Sikh); (2) the specific ways an individual might live out this identity in often unpredictable ways; and (3) the intersection of social and political forces in place that create the discursive and institutional spaces within which individuals would make their identity claims. That is, we need to address identities with all three approaches laid out above. Bearing these factors in mind helped us to reflect critically about why some individuals might be freer to explore, enact, or entertain certain identities in certain institutions (hospitals in Vancouver or London, for example) than others. From a practical perspective, this analysis helps to identify more clearly how to alter our institutions, or critically observe our public discourses, so that healthcare services are more inclusive.

COMPLICATING RELIGIOUS IDENTITIES WITH PARTICIPANT ACCOUNTS

With that groundwork laid, we present the ways that religious identities, as social constructions, were presented, negotiated, and transgressed for the individuals within our study. Because identities are social constructions, they do not exist within vacuums and are often a part of intersectional identities that include, for example, gender, ethnicity, culture, class, and sexuality. Studies of intersectionality (Collins 1990; Crenshaw 1989; hooks 1984) offer depth to our position that when religious identities were examined from a lived perspective, they cannot be understood in sui generis ways alone. When analyzing our data we were interested in, for example, when national, ethnic, or gender identities trump religious identities, or vice versa. Intersectionality also informs our approach to uncover how social and institutional structures make some identities more vulnerable and others privileged (Crenshaw 2016; Dhamoon and Hankivsky 2011). Hence prayer is a practice that enabled us to see the boundedness and fluidity of religious identities in these contexts.

The Social Relations of Prayer and the Presence of Sui Generis Identities

As we argued in the introduction to this chapter, there is an expectation that we can find coherent ethical, practical, and theological norms within the world religions approach. Following a sui generis approach to religious identities, there were multiple examples of people praying in expected ways and with expected people. At one of our London sites, where a multi-faith model of chaplaincy was principally operative (see chapter 5), we heard about, for example, Muslims praying with Muslims, Pagans praying with Pagans, and Catholics praying with Catholics. Ezra, a Jewish chaplain there stated, "I'm only in touch with Jewish patients."

Ezra's ability to know who was Jewish was predicated upon the completion of an intake survey (admission form) at the time of entry to hospital. Admission to hospital for patients and their families and friends is usually an uncertain time and, for some, a frightening experience. Under such circumstances of vulnerability or "precariousness" (Drescher 2016), religious identities may be evoked even if they have lain dormant for a period of time. It is not uncommon for people who rarely pray at other times to want to pray when faced with difficult circumstances, and they often draw upon memories of the tradition in which they were brought up to do so. Martha, a healthcare professional in London, explained: "Often, as we know, when people are coming towards the very end of their life … they just come back … it's back to home. For me, that's the way I understand it. It's back to home, back to what was it like to be a child, when did I feel safe, when did I feel comfort, what were all those rites of passage."

Whilst prayer may thus be welcomed, one of the difficulties the chaplains faced in responding to patients' spiritual needs was that it could be difficult to find out patients' religious affiliation. Although the intake clerk normally asked patients to state their religion, the options available to self-identify were broad and did not indicate denominational or cultural differences, and sometimes the admissions clerk at intake was inconsistent in asking this question. Religious studies scholar Jagbir Jhutti-Johal (2013) notes this situation for Sikhs in palliative care, whilst sociologist of religion Abby Day (2011) critiques the limitations of identity categories more generally. A chaplain, for example, could be left to determine between types of "no religion" and find out if people held some type of affiliation (such as belonging to the Humanist Association or the Secular Society), or if they were simply indifferent to religion. Annalise, a Vancouver chaplain, confirmed this ambiguity: "On the admission record there's a question about religion. And it often is left 'other' or 'unknown' or 'none'. And I think it was because there was some pushback about the question being asked by the intake person [admission clerk], so that was a big kafuffle many years ago. I'll find out they're Christian or they're Hindu or they're Sikh and it's like, we could have been supporting them. When it says 'none' or 'unknown', I don't take that as an official word." Even when information was accurately recorded, if direct referrals were not made, the chaplains could still be left having to do some detective work to establish a patient's affiliation. Consequently, some chaplains have suggested relying on clues such as the patient's dietary requests, objects around the patient's bed, patient names, and points in conversation, to work out whether and how to proceed with prayers. Alternatively, chaplains spoke about making themselves visible on the ward, as part of a proactive program to visit every ward, every week, and hoping that people who needed them would ask. Amelio, a chaplain in London, described the unreliability of the intake forms for accessing religious identities and the need to be accessible in other ways: "My main purpose on the wards is to be visible because yes, some are declaring they are Catholic in their admission. But most of the patients don't declare that they're Catholic. So my visibility means they will call me if they need to." A family member in Vancouver, Edna, also highlighted how access to chaplains often came through this visibility: "And it was nice because the lady came and she said, 'I'm the spiritual care. Do you have any faith-based beliefs or supports?' I said 'Actually yes I do. I could do with a prayer right now.'"

Healthcare staff, particularly nurses, also play an important role in this deciphering work. Luis, another chaplain in London, spoke about his presence on hospital wards as an entry point to referrals, but further described how he often found out who needed him from the nurses on the ward who determined that the patient was, for example, Catholic and needs a Catholic chaplain. Berna (chaplain, London) also discussed how conversations with nurses within the healthcare setting were important in determining who "might need my service." Similarly, Mohamed, a chaplain in London, discussed how the admission form was important, but even more so it was the "information taken by the staff on the ward [the healthcare staff], that will help us to identify what we are supposed to do." Emma, a healthcare professional in London, emphasized that there was a real difficulty for patients to express an identity when within the healthcare setting: "I don't feel like people really are able to express it in the way that they probably would want to express it," and thus it was difficult to determine who needed spiritual support. Once a tangible request for prayer was made, Zara (healthcare professional, London) explained that they as healthcare professionals can help organize space for patients and families to pray, to call in their faith leader, or "have somebody from the chaplaincy go and visit." In fact, Paresh (healthcare professional, London) explained that often, when patients for whom religion is important need support they will ask the nursing staff and the nursing staff will refer to the chaplain. When relying on healthcare professionals or others to interpret religious identity, bias can seep in. This was evidenced when one of our research team discussed spiritual care support services with a healthcare professional (Liam) in Vancouver.

> LIAM: Most patients here identify as Christian ... so we do celebrate: we put up the Christmas and Easter and sort of those things. I don't think we make a point of asking people what denomination they belong to. We don't seek out that information. Maybe it's something we should do. I don't know.
> RESEARCHER: When you say most of the clients are Christian, is this information that they give up freely in their conversations with you?
> LIAM: It's an assumption that I'm making from the operation of the clinic. But we don't formally collect that data, so I don't know what percentage are Christian.

The difficulty with chaplains and healthcare professionals deciphering people's religious identity was that patients of minority faiths might have gone unseen. Since the systems and processes in place to access religious identities within our research sites seldom captured the nuances of religious identities, did not always get asked, or could be biased in favour of majoritarian religions, we posited that some individuals were likely left without access to religious supports and practices in healthcare institutions.

When chaplains in London knew a patient's religion, they typically arranged for a chaplain of the same faith to attend to any needs that might arise. While we will see below how sometimes the more informal requests or experiences led to people praying across religious traditions, recognition of a shared religious (or cultural) identity, particularly as they were marked out in formal prayers, was a way of making a connection with patients, evoking a sense of the familiar and providing comfort. One diary entry from Paul, a Catholic chaplain in London, for example, recorded how he had spoken to an elderly Catholic patient about the "Irish faith family traditions" that they both knew, which led them to saying the rosary together.

An advantage of chaplains working within their own tradition was that they had knowledge of the prayers most likely to be familiar to patients, even if the patient had lapsed in practice. They also had the knowledge and dexterity to modify traditional prayer practices to meet patients' needs where appropriate. Thus Ali, a Muslim chaplain in London, described how he would teach a bed-bound Muslim who could not get to a mosque or assume the normal prayer positions, how these conventions could be adapted to current circumstances: "You can stay in your bed. If you can't move your head, fine. If you can't move your head, just say it with your eye. You can pray with your eye."

Frances, a chaplain in Vancouver, explained that even though their chaplaincy model was a generic one that enabled them to support people from all faith traditions, there were still limits. In her research diary, she described an interaction that she had with an Indigenous family where she facilitated access to the First Nations sacred space, an Indigenous elder, and the materials for smudging. In describing the smudging ceremony, she explained, "I had tears coming down my face. I felt that the young were well cared for. I could never have cared for their spiritual well-being as well as their *own* [emphasis ours] people were able to do it. I could only provide the opportunity for them to do this [providing the quiet space, privacy, and time to be together in smudging and prayer]." A sui generis approach to religious identities here led to what Cadge and Sigelow (2013) refer to as "matching," where the Indigenous identity of the elder matched that of the family. So, on the one hand, sometimes the boundaries of religious identity remained in place, which could offer more meaningful connections, as in the above examples. On the other hand, sometimes the boundaries of religious identity were challenged and crossed in the everyday, lived experiences of prayer in healthcare settings. We turn to such examples now.

The Social Relations of Prayer and the Flexibility of Lived Identities

While a sui generis framework of religion enabled chaplains to walk alongside patients and families who shared their faith tradition, participants were often in situations where such identities were not shared, or where patients might see or identify the chaplain but presume that they have been or will be ostracized from their religion of origin because of their life choices and identities made complicated by intersecting social structures. Prayer was a window on how religion as lived was more complicated in the diverse contexts of our hospital sites. It was not uncommon for participants to transgress expectations of religious identities in the enactment of prayer. In other words, when participants did not match or share a faith tradition, or did not feel comfortable doing so, they employed other strategies to maintain or cross boundaries while respecting difference. As Jane asserted, "When I pray with people, they pray with me, we are crossing boundaries. It's not like anything else because prayer crosses so much. It crosses people's lives. It crosses faith traditions, religions." Her description evoked lived encounters and the process involved in finding mutual meaning in prayer rituals or practices shared across religious cultures. By engaging in what Cadge and Sigelow (2013, 148) would call "neutralizing difference," the interfaith pray-ers engaged in prayer practices with the intention not to find commonalities between religious traditions, nor view religious difference positively, but simply to allow space for different traditions to co-exist. Wendy, a chaplain in London, described how she had lit a candle in the chapel, and a Hindu mother took the heat from the candle to bless her child. The chaplain then gave her own blessing. Others practised "minimizing of difference," where they looked to find mutual meanings in prayer rituals or practices that were shared across religious cultures. An Orthodox chaplain listed a range of things that his tradition had in common with others: "For Hindus, the Ganges is like baptism. Light for them is hope and we do the same with candles. We both have respect for our elders." That mutual meanings found in traditions and prayers do not, however, mean that the *same* meanings are found by the patient and chaplain. Mona (chaplain, London), for example, recognized that people prayed in their own way and was relaxed with the idea that somebody might want to "hug trees" because within the tree they saw their God. Minimizing difference therefore ran the risk of prayers being misinterpreted but meant that faith identities were more often uncompromised and navigated harmoniously.

These kinds of navigations were facilitated by a generic model of chaplaincy outlined in chapter 5. Because chaplains under this model were often assigned to units rather than religions, prayer across religious identities was a norm rather than an exception. As one chaplain, proclaimed, "We don't care whether it's Catholic or Protestant or Sikh or whatever. If they call us, we're going to go." Curtis described experiences of praying with individuals from other religious traditions, in what Cadge and Sigelow refer to as "code switching" (2013, 148), explaining that they simply adjusted their language and allowed the individuals to lead them in the kind of prayer that would be meaningful to them. He explained how these experiences, while potentially awkward and strange, were in reality easily negotiated in the moment of prayer: "If I'm dealing with people who have a different belief system, I often find that there's a charity and expansiveness on their part. I remember walking into a room. I was going to go visit a patient, but the patient had been discharged and someone else was in the bed. I was going to excuse myself and said, 'I came in, because I had promised so-and-so that I would pray with them before they got discharged but I guess they got discharged early.' And they said, 'Oh you were going to pray? Well, we're Baha'i. We'd love to have you pray with us.' They could see my awkwardness and they said, 'You can pray in the name of Jesus. We're fine with that.'" While the multi-faith dynamic of the mixed models present at London sites most often paired chaplains with patients who shared their faith tradition, they also engaged in prayer with patients who were not on their list, as part of the more generic approach to chaplaincy that was employed, especially by on-call chaplains and through regular ward rounds. As Mona explained, "Even if it was a non-Muslim ... I could tender a prayer for them. Sometimes I'll see older Caribbean women. Then my prayer will be to God, and not to Jesus Christ; that will be the difference. I will pray for goodness for them." Another dynamic was at play here, in that Mona foregrounded their shared gender and ethnicity, which allowed prayer to happen. Points of connection apart from religion were also present when Frida, a Christian chaplain in London, undertaking a "generic" ward round, described an occasion when a Muslim woman wanted her to pray with her in preference to a male imam. At first Frida hesitated because she was not a Muslim and did not want to get herself or the patient "into trouble." Once she was reassured that the patient was happy to go ahead despite their religious differences, she prayed an informal prayer for the patient. Similar to Mona, what mattered in the lived encounter was Frida's identity as a woman, not necessarily an identity as "Muslim" or "Christian." In these examples, the concept of intersectionality can reveal how social structures such as gender enable prayer encounters.

The Social Relations of Prayer
and the Critique Offered by Intersectionality

Studies of intersectionality demonstrate how limits set up by social structures such as race, gender, and class can be transgressed by individual acts of agency (Brah and Phoenix 2009; Collins 1990; Crenshaw 1989). Here we address the ways in which identities were sometimes bounded by social structures or institutional approaches to identity. That is, we explore how webs of social and political forces created the discursive and institutional spaces within which participants made identity claims and in which prayer practices were consequently affected.

We heard how participants chose to foreground or hide their religious identities because of social and political factors (in reality or in perception). According to Werbner (2010), identity often emerges when in conflict, when challenged, or when politicized. In the past twenty years, and especially after the events of 11 September 2001, Muslim identities have become highly politicized. We saw evidence of this from comments that Laura, an administrator in Vancouver, shared about Muslim patients hesitant to provide their religious identities on the site's admission form: "For example, we can change the religious answers of the patient if not correct, or if the patient agrees that it can be changed. Some patients don't want to tell who they are. Like when it was an anniversary of 9/11, I had several Muslim patients who wanted to say that they were not Muslim. So I respected that." Laura went on to explain that by not claiming their Muslim identities, patients may not have been supported in certain aspects of their religious practice. For example, the kitchen would not know that they might require specific dietary provisions, and chaplains might not know that they would like access to prayer space. In contexts such as North America and Europe, where there has been a rise in Islamophobia since 9/11 and the more recent 2014 refugee crisis (Allen 2010; Davis and Zarkov 2017), Muslim identities are not only seen as monolithic and all-encompassing for those who hold one, but also are racialized and demonized. To resist essentialism and discrimination, the Muslim patients described by Laura chose to conceal their religious identities.

As noted, structures of gender intersected with the social relations of prayer. In London, Berna, a female chaplain who holds a racialized identity, described a situation where a white, male, Catholic priest was a patient in the hospital. She came to pray with this man, and he refused. She explained that he did not want a multi-faith encounter (even though she was Catholic herself), and that he held a specific idea of what a Catholic chaplain should look like: "He knows men but not women.... I've learned there is no rush to see a reverend father who is on the ward." We see here how gender and power affected this meeting, but racialization might also underlie the priest's response to Berna offering to pray for him. Historically, "Christianity has been racialized through its association with whiteness" (Joshi 2006, 212). Hence racialization operates in tandem with religion in both overt and covert ways. While gender was an aspect of her identity perceived as restrictive to a mutual religious identity, racialization could also limit acts of giving and receiving prayer. From an intersectional perspective, historical patriarchy and colonialism operated in the background to structure this encounter.

These types of interactions revealed individuals' assumptions about what a given identity means and who has the right to claim that identity. Tara, a healthcare professional, described her response to a patient with substance addiction who told her he was a Christian: "I was blown away, and this is a horrible thought to have: 'How can an addict be a Christian?'... I've never assumed the clients here to be Christian, or of any faith background, because they're coming here for the drug ... and that's an idol." Here we see how certain identities are assumed to be out of the realm of "Christian" identity. The participant reveals a bounded understanding of what Christian qua Christian identity "must" be (i.e., that one cannot have idols and be a Christian). When face-to-face with someone who transgressed her ideas of Christian identity, she had to adjust her perspective.

Tara later brought sexuality into the conversation, demonstrating her advocacy on behalf of the LGBTQIA community as she told of a situation in which she prayed with a gay man. At the same time that she critiqued religion's "hate on the LGBT community forever," she valued the integration of spirituality into healthcare to the extent that it was important to her clients. She understood, then, the historical and contemporary structuring of social exclusion, yet herself showed agency in mitigating how these structures would affect her and her clients in the religiously affiliated organization in which she worked. Ersi, another healthcare professional, also conveyed that intersecting structures of sexual and religious inequalities can affect religious and gay individuals and their access and openness to spiritual care and prayer. She explained how many of the gay individuals she worked with had a hard time reconciling their spirituality with their sexuality and generally avoided spiritual practices because of it. Capturing this tension, she cogently observed that they were discriminated against for their sexuality in their religious lives, and for their religiosity in their sexual lives (also see El-Tayeb 2012; Yip 2000, 2003) (see chapter 6). In the above examples, we see how religious identities and the offering and receiving of prayer were complicated by structures of race, gender, class, and sexuality. Intersectionality makes visible how structures can oppress but also how they can be resisted by agential acts. This agency contributed to holding space for prayer and thereby transgressed the social and institutional structures that undergirded normative constructions associated with sexism, racism, classism, and homophobia.

At the beginning of this chapter we posed the question, "What do we have in mind when we say Paresh is a Sikh or Grace a Christian?" Using our three-fold framework allowed us to understand our participants' experiences; for example, at one level Paresh and Grace were affiliating themselves to religious traditions recognized from a sui generis world religion perspective to be associated with a particular set of beliefs, practices, and behavioural norms. This perspective provided health- and spiritual-care providers with a framework upon which to plan and offer provision of prayer spaces and liturgies, and so forth. But we also saw that from a lived religion perspective, identities were not bound and prescriptive. Rather, personal preferences, individual biographies, and competing cultural norms all came into play such that prayer transgressed boundaries to find points of commonality and shared understanding that might otherwise have been missed. Prayer was transgressive as it both affirmed and transcended religious identities and norms, and opened individuals up to new ways of engaging with others. Beyond this, we found that organizational processes could serve to limit and delineate religious identities claimed and supported in the healthcare setting. An intersectional reading helped to uncover assumptions (such as middle-class views on spirituality) and structures (such as patriarchy and racism) that were doing their work, just below the surface. How prayer is worked out at the nexus of sui generis understandings, the realities of lived religion, and the constraints of institutional limits and social structures is at the heart of the social relations of prayer. The materiality of prayer, the focus of the next chapter, also engages with influences on the social relations of prayer, specifically material culture, embodiment, and the senses.

When Some "Body" Prays:
Materiality and the Senses in Prayer

Rachel Brown and Melania Calestani

You've got the prayer where you speak to God, you bow your head, put your hands together and you pray.

Lata and Joseph, citizens, London

I always look at prayer as breathing. I pray whenever I breathe.

Ronald, chaplain, Vancouver

With these comments, our participants Lata, Joseph, and Ronald reflected that the sacred is made real and present through the body and material objects. In this chapter we examine what things, objects, and bodies do. This is in line with the material turn in the study of religion whereby "religion [and prayer] is unable to do without things, places, or bodies, nor may it operate without theories about materiality" (Meyer et al. 2010, 210). Material things are exchanged and circulated, bearing values and power that structure human relations and the social relations of prayer (Olsen 2003). Within biomedical contexts, bodies are an intimate focus. In our study, prayer could transgress clinical settings in intimate ways where it was not the vulnerability of the physical body that one confronted but that of the soul and spirit. Biomedicine is critiqued for only looking after the body, but prayer counters that tendency, intervening via the bodily and the material sense and not for the sake of the body only. In what follows, we capture these aspects through prayer as expressed and embodied through material culture, embodiment, and the senses.

MATERIAL CULTURE AND PRAYER

In our research we noted that prayer in healthcare could be facilitated by the use of specific objects and religious artifacts, which thereby came to embody a mediatory role with the transcendent (Espírito Santo and Tassi 2013). These objects were not simply mediators or projectors of social and cosmological relations, but such artifacts could (re)produce these relations through their circulation, motion, aesthetic proprieties and mutability, and embeddedness in social life (Espírito Santo and Tassi 2013). Our participants discussed physical objects, such as prayer beads, prayer mats, head scarves, and turbans. Zara, a healthcare professional in London, talked about the importance of prayer bags: "We used to have some volunteers who came on a regular basis and gave out little prayer bags with some prayers and things. On many occasions, I also received one of these, which I thought was sweet and nice. It helps you to connect spiritually because you feel like there is somebody religious, nice, caring, kind, and thinking of you." In this we saw an example of what sociologist Elizabeth Drescher (2016, 171) has defined as "contingent vulnerability." In Drescher's work, the concept of contingent vulnerability in relation to prayer is what sets prayer apart. It is the idea that people engage in prayer because of its ability to express something more than surface concern. Saying you will pray for someone, or in this case, providing prayer bags, reflects a deeper level of concern than saying, "I'm thinking of you." When you say you are praying for someone, Drescher argues that this reflects the idea "that your sense of security, safety, and health is connected to mine, at least emotionally" (as quoted in Roychoudhuri 2015, n.p.). Offering to pray for someone is a way of narrating that fact. The offering or giving of prayer through material objects can be viewed as an intimate act that goes beyond a typical routine health check by a nurse or doctor. It crosses into the realm of the sacred. It is a social act, traversing the profane of the clinical setting to involve the transcendent.

Material religious objects transgress the biomedical and are imbued with power. Socio-cultural sociologist Arjun Appadurai (1994) has shown that material things have a social life, and their circulation has a symbolic meaning in terms of power relations and human interactions. Andreas, a chaplain (Vancouver) mused, "Why do you give to the Catholic patients rosaries for free, and to the Muslim patients you don't give beads for free?" This reflected a fair point as, in one site,

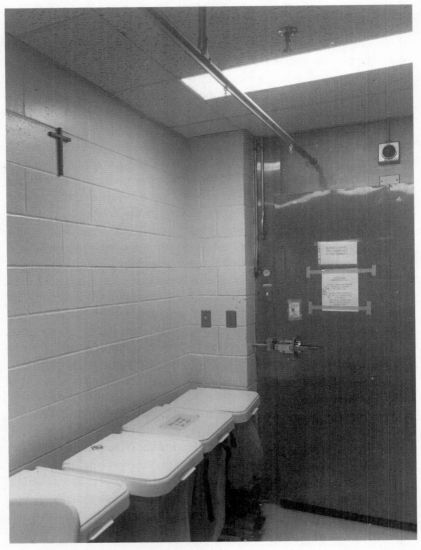

8.1 Crosses in institutional spaces

Bibles, New Testaments, the Quran, and Gita were given free. Muslim beads were few and tended to go quickly. Andreas's quote highlighted the power and privilege attached to these objects. His quote inferred a priority was given to Christians and to the specific material culture necessary to engage in certain prayer practices, such as rosary beads. Power was attached to these objects that were made available to some and not to others. As shown in chapter 3, access to space symbolized power relations, and this was also the case with access to certain material objects, which further reflected religious histories and social hierarchies.

Similarly a Hindu-Christian couple (Lata and Joseph) raised the issue that there were not enough Hindu objects and images in the hospital. They explained that specific objects constitute the tapestry of the material culture of their prayer in Hinduism. Joseph said, "My wife will light the *Divo* [the divine flame]. She will use ghee or oil. She gets a little bit of cotton wool, that becomes the wick and she has something that holds it up. And then she will pray.... I find prayer to be a very interesting thing: it's our only link to connect to the Higher Being that exists, that no one can see." This participant suggested that prayer through the lighting of the divine flame was essential and the "only link" to connect to the Higher Being, and yet one would be hard pressed to find divine flames distributed around healthcare settings. In this we observed that some prayer practices were privileged through the material culture that was available in healthcare settings.

The visibility of Christian material culture at some of our research sites was expressed through the materiality of crosses, which one could find in each hospital room, often mounted above the doorways (see figure 8.1). We were told that the crosses had replaced earlier crucifixes about ten years ago, as a way to be more ecumenical. The visibility of the crosses nonetheless raised issues about the protection of religious belief, non-religious expressions, and different religions (Beaman, Steele, and Pringnitz 2018). Angela, an administrator in Vancouver, told us, "How does this setting influence spirituality? That's a really good question. I think on the one hand it lends legitimacy to spirituality. On the other hand, it leans toward Christianity. If I was someone coming into this setting, as a strong believer of another religion, I'm not sure how I would feel about all the crosses. I'm not sure how safe I would feel in talking about my own beliefs." This idea of safety could refer to how some users of a clinical setting might feel that because of the strong visibility of a majoritarian religion, other beliefs or faiths were unwelcome. There were times when crosses were taken down, either by request of a patient or family, or from a formally designated space for meditation. The staff member charged with overseeing the crosses as part of her portfolio described the taking down and putting up of crosses as an "informal practice. If somebody is disturbed by the cross, we take it down. What happens is the cross goes to the nursing station, put in a drawer, and people forget to put it back up, and then it's lost. Somebody will eventually say to me, 'We're missing eight crosses up here.'" There was both an intentional messaging and a fluidity of presence of the crosses within religiously affiliated healthcare organizations. They were not permanently fixed on walls and they came and went on the basis of users' preferences. The inhabiting of clinical spaces and the spaces of faith within them were often negotiated through material culture, not only among different faith groups and those of no affiliation, but also with management, staff, and patients, as our participant explained, signalling important forms of agency among different user groups. The privileging of certain religious identities, discussed in chapter 7, was enacted through these material objects.

The privilege given to Indigenous prayer in a First Nations sacred space provided a contrast to the highly visible Christian material culture described at some of our Vancouver sites (see chapter 3). In this case, a separate space demonstrating Indigenous rights and the process of reconciliation was set aside and embraced in this healthcare context. This reflected Canada's 2015 Truth and Reconciliation Commission's Call to Action 22: "We call upon those who can effect change within the Canadian healthcare system to recognize the value of Aboriginal healing practices in collaboration with Aboriginal healers and Elders where requested by Aboriginal patients" (TRC Calls to Action 2015). At many of our Vancouver sites, material culture was deeply embedded, especially within one First Nations sacred space. The fabric of the prayer ribbons, the stones and cedar bows, the sage for smudging, the objects for traditional tea, and the drum for healing circles all structured interactions and relations of prayer that tied together material and immaterial sacred worlds (see figure 8.2).

In clinical contexts that may be perceived as anaesthetized or sterile, some of our participants felt a need to express their identity through religious artifacts, but also through religious pieces of clothing. Anthropologist Emma Tarlo (2007) writes about the significance of dress as a visible indicator of multicultural difference. Religious pieces of clothing helped to facilitate prayer for some and yet were an obstacle for others. Thomas, a Vancouver chaplain, told us, "Dog collars [clerical collars] these days can be much less of an open [door] and much more of a deterrent for some people.... Yet I find that I don't lack ability or opportunity to pray without a dog collar on."

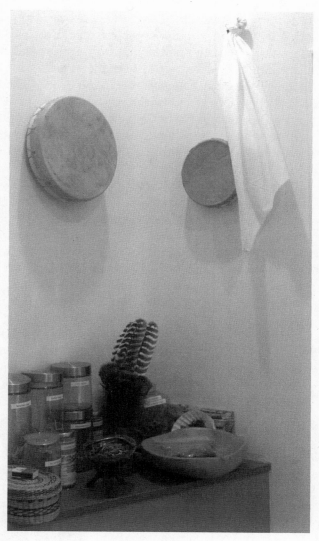

8.2 Material culture in a First Nations sacred space

Chaplains at our London sites wore clothing representative of their faith traditions. In Vancouver, only the Catholic priests wore a clerical collar. At one site where religious garments were the norm for most of the chaplains, Hannah, a London chaplain who did not come from a tradition with identifiable clerical clothing, told us that "because we don't wear special clothes, the nursing staff will not necessarily respond to us the way that they would to somebody who was dressed in the recognizable uniform of clergy." She described a situation where she attended to a patient and family, where the family were not getting what they needed for their loved one. She stated, "If I had a dog collar they [the nursing staff] wouldn't have ignored me." These examples revealed the clerical garb as an obstacle on the one hand and an entry point on the other hand. In both cases, religious clothing was imbued with power to bring religion and religious authority into the most intimate healthcare encounters. These examples further highlighted the material working out of the liminality of chaplains as discussed in chapter 5.

Beyond questions of power and offence, pieces of clothing that symbolized identity could facilitate prayer practices. Mona (chaplain, London) recalled an episode with a Muslim patient who did not have a head scarf and was not comfortable seeing the imam without one. She told us, "I took one of the nurses' aprons and made a head scarf for her and then the imam could come in." In this encounter, the use of an apron was innovative and responsive to the centrality of specific garments needed for prayer, and as such evidences that faith is entangled with materiality that is simultaneously gendered. Another example was provided by Zara, who talked about a Sikh patient affected by stroke: "The stroke had affected his hand. He couldn't control his turban and he felt dependent on other people to help him organize his image. His turban is part of his religion. I felt when he said to me, 'Nurse,' he inferred, 'do you realize how much this has affected me and the fact that I feel lopsided with my turban?'" The turban can be particularly significant for some Sikhs in terms of identity, and this narrative indicated how the patient could have felt incomplete when unable to independently arrange it. These two examples of covering one's head expose dynamics of how deeply personal gender and religious relations can be. The vulnerabilities of illness and the homogenizing tendencies of healthcare contexts can leave patients dependent on the religious literacy of health professionals (Dinham and Francis 2015). The volunteer and the nurse recognized the importance of religious clothing to the practices of their patients' faith, and, through their actions, ensured they were respected. These intimate acts heeded the cultural contexts that informed the patients' everyday experiences of their bodies and that extended beyond biomedical functioning.

Other material obstacles to prayer showed up at our sites. We saw this in the provision of washing facilities for patients who wanted to prepare themselves for prayers. For many people of varying religious backgrounds (specifically Muslims and Sikhs in our data), there is an emphasis on coming to prayer in a state of cleanliness. Ali, a chaplain, explained the impact of this specific obstacle on Muslim prayer: "Usually a prayer in Islam needs a lot of rules.... Your body must be clean, and before you pray you must do ablution, you must do the washing ... [but] patients cannot do ablution. Some of them are carrying the bag for urine and they want to pray. They feel the only way to they can be close to God is through prayer. So they call me, and I must explain to them how they can do the prayer." Mona described many options available to patients if there were no cleaning facilities present and they wanted to pray. Whether it was using a stone, dust, sand, or some other natural substance, there were ways to move beyond the obstacle of not having water present to conduct one's ablutions. She explained "dry ablution" or *tayammum*,[1] as follows: "God will answer even if you rub your hand on the clean sheets. It's a practicality.... If you haven't got the stone and you need to pray, just rub your hand on the sheet. God will accept. Well, we pray God will accept it because you haven't got any other means." The sacred and cleansed body were significant to prayer, but sometimes the body itself could be an obstacle to prayer, particularly in a medical context when confronted with disease and machines that prevent fluid expression of physical bodies. Religious literacy was conveyed by the imam and volunteer. Their guidance and suggestions demonstrated the flexibility of bodies and rituals to transgress material and bodily boundaries so that residents' and patients' prayer practices were honoured. In the next section, we analyze this notion of embodiment in more detail, weaving in the narratives of our participants.

DEALING WITH THE BODY

The body has long been a significant site for religion. Embodiment draws attention to the body as a means of "perceptual experience and mode of presence and engagement in the world" (Csordas 1994, 12). Embodying religious practice and prayer through holding religious artifacts, wearing religious pieces of clothing, engaging in cleansing rituals, along with kneeling, dancing, praying, singing, or bowing can be essential to belief (Morgan 2012). The body becomes a semiotic resource (Corwin 2012). Tulio (chaplain, Vancouver) described bowing in *namaste* as an embodied action through which he created a sacred space with an elderly Hindu gentleman (see chapter 7). Others discussed walking when describing moments of prayer, with Martin (chaplain) stating that "this is a viable prayer, putting one step in front of another." Prayer required our participants to engage not only with their own bodies, but also with those of others. Tulio explained, "I'm called to attend to the body constantly.... I think it's a wonderful opportunity for caregivers, not just spiritual caregivers, to tend to the body. We are forced by various bodily circumstances to be more attentive to our residents and their bodies. Most are in wheelchairs, for instance. We have to decide, are we going to stand and hover over them or will we actually get down in our bodies and be at the same level as they are?" Embodied attunement to the physical position of oneself and another happened with patients who were alive, and with those who had died. Jane (chaplain, Vancouver) told us, "Our role [as chaplains] is to bring the body from the morgue to the viewing room. If there's tidying up to be done, which often there is, to set up the body in such a way that it's as nice as you can [make it] ... it's very sacred and very special." Through these accounts we observed that one's own body and other people's bodies were essential for the enactment of prayer, and that these bodies contributed to the creation of sacred spaces. Where one no longer had control over one's own body (e.g., when wheelchair bound or in death), the body of another became an essential extension into the sacred. In clinical settings, patients' bodies were both subject to intimate interactions and kept at an analytical distance. When attuned to the sacred, meetings between patients and chaplains and spiritual care volunteers in medical contexts crossed into a space that was aware of the clinical and yet became an encounter set apart because of prayer.

The social relations of prayer that emerged from our participants' narratives are evocative of sociologist Yasmin Gunaratnam's (2013) work on how care happens in moments of interaction and negotiation at the borders of bodies, and of life and death. She writes about how bodies may create chaotic moments of hybridity and liminality (Gunaratnam 2014), which may imply different expectations when it comes to care and, in this case, end-of-life care. In particular, she writes, "These are marginal times and places, marked by a breakdown and crisis in the social; everything is up in the air, events unfurl unpredictably, moment-by-moment; decisions could go either way. Three key and intersecting layers of this rich analysis are relevant to hybridity at times of transnational and debilitated dying, when the borders between the socio-cultural, the body and affect, the present and the past can produce nested transitional states" (2014, 76). She names these layers of analysis as (1) holding together event and structure; (2) opening up to affectivity; and (3) giving attention to the socio-cultural infusing of life's transitional moments. In line with Gunaratnam's work, our participants engaged in narratives about moments of tension in healthcare settings, especially when the care provided for the body did not mirror the expectation of family members. Hannah talked about her experience with a Pagan family: "The woman died at two in the morning and the family wanted to take their mother's body home quickly to have a home wake. They had organized the burial in advance because they knew their mother was dying. However, healthcare staff told the family to go home and come back three days later for the body. The family said 'no,' they wanted to take the body the same day because they wanted a very quick burial in accordance with their religious views. And they had actually staged a stakeout. They locked themselves into the room with their mother's body and they refused to go." The family's response in the crisis moments between death and the wake demonstrated the chaotic, liminal spaces that were difficult to negotiate for the patient's family and the healthcare providers. Hannah drew attention to this upheaval and transitional moment because of the heightened invisibility of Pagan beliefs in this particular situation: "The family knew that this was done regularly for Jewish and Muslim bodies, that they are released quickly by the hospital. The sanctity of the body and that it has to return to the earth is believed by many Pagans. There's the embodied spirituality and the coming to terms with the cycles of life. Engaging with the body is a central principle." The sanctity of the body and yet the relative invisibility of the Pagan belief system (compared to other religions) left this family in a vulnerable place. This case brought to light institutional healthcare policy on release of the body and the need to accommodate all faith and belief perspectives. When religion is read on the body, many come to expect visible markers (see Goffman 1963 on stigma and the role of bodily marks in exposing moral status). This is not always the case, raising the point of how Wiccans, Pagans, Humanists, and other non-religious individuals and groups embody their beliefs.

The embodied nature of clinical work itself, and the focus on the secularized biomedical work of the body, could act as a further obstacle to prayer. Although it is more than twenty-five years since anthropologist Margaret Lock (1993) suggested that there has been a demise of the idea of a biomedical body that is fixed in time and space, our participants continued to perceive and experience clinical settings as those that fix the physical body as the norm. Kirstie, a citizen, described her situation: "The hospital is too focused on the physical body, which makes it hard to engage the spiritual. You're tired. The atmosphere is not conducive to prayer, or to feeling particularly alive spiritually. It is a physical emphasis. The focus is on your body, not on your soul." In her experience, this lack of attention to the spiritual body, and the emphasis on the physical body, meant that senses and materiality that were significant to prayer could be sidelined. Social, cultural, and religious identities could be missed. Chaplains shared similar perspectives. Jane (chaplain, Vancouver) described this imbalance: "In the middle of prayer, somebody coming in with the lunch tray and putting it down. You think, 'Just allow this moment to happen.' It would be as if a nurse had somebody half stripped naked and was giving them an injection in their backside. Would the person still come in and leave the lunch tray? I don't know if they would." Jane recounted the vulnerability of prayer, such that the person bringing in a lunch tray contributed to the creation of borders that could limit prayer from happening. Bedsides became sites of interaction and negotiation between different social actors and categories of people (chaplains, faith leaders, healthcare professionals, and family members). Bodies may then be constructed as sacred entities by some individuals, but also concurrently as institutional sites of surveillance by others such as healthcare professionals focused on feeding and treating the body (Smith 2012). Medical sociologist David Armstrong (1983, 1995) wrote that the twentieth century marked a shift in the clinical gaze, from a focus on the interior of the body, to a focus that both explored the body in relation to its exterior and to the collective body. He went on to describe this new mechanism of power as "surveillance medicine" (Armstrong 1995; see also Foucault [1973] 2003; Lock 1993). Clinical settings emphasize the body in ways that other research sites would not, creating medicalized bodies that are surveilled by ethical systems, internationalized protocols, and evidence-based practices. As our data on prayer demonstrated, bodies could transgress institutional and medical power, by testing and bridging between clinical, institutional, and spiritual priorities.

SENSING PRAYER

When we think about the body, we cannot avoid connecting embodiment with the senses, which influence the way we construct our worlds. Anthropologist David Howes (2015, 153) suggests that the term *sense* includes and expresses "both sensation *and* signification, feeling *and* meaning in its spectrum of referents. To 'sense the world' is, therefore, both to register it through the senses and to imbue those registrations with significance." Sociologist Pierre Bourdieu (1977, 24) also contends that our senses, both physical and social, are involved in remembering and embodying practices. The engagement of the senses, whether intentional or not, was a reality that inevitably affected the performance of prayer by patients, residents, staff, and others in healthcare settings. Katrina, a healthcare professional in Vancouver, reflected on the importance of all the senses in her experiences of prayer: "Opening to [the] present, and not just being stuck in the past or the future but being where I am and noticing my senses and noticing my body and noticing the people around me. When I am in that place, I feel more authentic in praying or interacting with other people." For many, senses are central to any experience or discussion of religion. Anthropologist of religion Birgit Meyer writes that religion should be seen as "sensational forms" (2006, 2009), in that the transcendental is rendered sensible (2006). When considering practices such as prayer, which are often imbued with transcendent significance, the senses played a central role in making that transcendent experience imminent, sometimes facilitating the experience and sometimes hindering it.

Sight and Sound

In this section we explore the impact of the senses on prayer practices and consequently on the social relations of prayer that emerged from our data. We begin with a discussion of sight and sound. Sight enables one to see and to be seen. One can look at or look away. Rosa, a healthcare professional, described how sight could help some people engage with spiritual practices: "Many people are visual, so I think people who may not really have a prayerful practice or a spiritual communion might find it helpful to write it [prayer] down or to hang it up. If seeing it doesn't make the prayer more relevant to you, you can take it down or you can just allow the staff to take it down." The sight of crosses around healthcare settings in Vancouver, described above, was another example of how sight might facilitate or hinder prayer, depending on individuals' religious identity and their view of religious symbols. Similarly, the arts (e.g., paintings, photography, and sculpture) had a notable impact on sight and experiences of prayer at our field sites (see chapter 9). Viewing a piece of art could conjure spiritual insights, such as a way of seeing one's situation and circumstances anew.

Sound contributed to the construction of clinical spaces. What was heard on a hospital ward could generate distance and intimacy between staff, patients, and families. Sometimes the sound of individual or collective prayers could repel, disquiet, and draw one near. Sound was a sense that facilitated, or not, the act of prayer in healthcare contexts. As an example of an auditory angle on prayer, some of the Vancouver sites used to broadcast morning prayers over the intercom, but they had been discontinued to create a more inclusive environment. Maryanne, an administrator in Vancouver, told us that she missed these morning prayers. Another example came from Berna (chaplain, London), who told us about the importance of using the body to communicate when patients are hard of hearing, especially in a busy and noisy hospital: "There's noise and nurses and doctors passing. That's another obstacle. We can't really [give] focus to prayer ... especially Catholic prayers ... because if there's no silence it's difficult to focus." The soundscapes of hospitals described by participants were not easily containable and inevitably transgressed clinical spaces, where patients, staff, and families could hear each other and be affected. Practices of prayer could be susceptible to aural limitations. Likewise, the sounds of prayer could be a sonic comfort to individuals and groups of patients and an imposition. Music was described as being conducive to experiences of prayer such as through a radio at the bedside or live classical noontime concerts held for hospital constituents (see chapter 9).

Taste and Smell

Taste also played a role in the daily enactment of prayer in healthcare settings. For some, especially for those who, because of context, were restricted in their traditional, religious, and cultural practices, food and the experience of taste could take up a central role in everyday practice. One might not be able to get to the cathedral to partake in the Eucharist, but one could still access communion in the healthcare setting. As Rinaldo (chaplain, Vancouver) said, "If I was a Catholic wanting to receive Mass or Holy Communion, but I couldn't, I would like somebody to bring me there." When people cannot be brought to Mass, hospital volunteers bring the "bread" sacrament to the patients, to their bedside, crossing physical boundaries so the patient can cross spiritual ones in the act of ingesting the Eucharist. This is reflective of work within religion and food studies that suggests that food, and the experience of ingesting familiar tastes, crosses boundaries of time and space (Brown 2017). Orthodox chaplains in both Vancouver and London explained that by taking the Eucharist to the patients on the wards, the wards became a place of prayer. It is the material elements of communion and the experience of ingesting those elements that transform the space into intimate, sacred, prayer-full space. Curtis (chaplain) explained, "With just a little bit of bread and water ... there is something about the ability to infuse objects with symbolic meaning ... to transcend the reality and connect with that which is beyond." As a food event, the Eucharist at the bedside could communicate healing and comfort. According to anthropologist David Sutton (2001, 83), the "food event evokes a whole world of family" and therefore creates a feeling of wholeness in the individual, a wholeness that is often threatened, or feels distant, when in healthcare settings (for more on prayer and the pursuit of wholeness, see chapter 6).

Like the other senses, smell could both facilitate and hinder prayer practices in the healthcare setting. Smell could affect prayer practices quite unintentionally, or it could be harnessed and used: materials to invoke the sense of smell could be used to facilitate prayer in the healthcare setting. Multiple participants discussed how the smells of hospitals could be a distraction to their interactions with patients, but they would "try to be composed and pray when I approach each patient" (Amelio, chaplain). A Muslim chaplain explained how urine and a dirty body conjured a strong negative sense of smell and thereby contributed to distance between him and the patient (Goffman 1963). Frida (chaplain, London) explained that the clinical smells of the hospital prevented her from pursuing her "calling" as a chaplain for a long time. The fact that scents could deter or enable prayer was made even more evident by Margaret (chaplain), who described a place particularly conducive to prayer: "It's [the corridor] very airy and it's very near the roof, because it's the fourth floor, and it's very open, and because it's not in a ward it's quite unstuffy and it's not smelly. One of the wards I go to is quite smelly. It's a moment of freshness." At our Vancouver sites, scent fused with material culture to facilitate specific prayer practices in a First Nations prayer space. Smudges, the ritual burning of aromatic and medicinal plants during prayers, played a central role in the prayer practices of First Nations patients and staff. Geographer Kathleen Wilson (2003) discusses how some First Nations individuals see smudges as essential to healing, and some also believe that their "prayers get offered up to the Creator through the smoke" (89). Liam, a healthcare professional in Vancouver, discussed this practice: "A couple of First Nations folks ... had done smudges, a spiritual practice for them and their connection to their spiritual traditions. They are doing it to help us and cleanse the space. That's a shared prayer." While the sense of smell could dissuade prayer, it could also aid in its practice and cross boundaries of religious affiliation, as observed in this case.

Touch and Intuition

The sense of touch was also discussed by our participants, as was intuition as a "sixth sense." Touch could create a moment of intimacy with another, letting patients know they were not alone in their experience of illness. Touch could also convey prayer. Ronald told us that a typical understanding of prayer was "holding someone's hand." Berna expressed positive emotions around prayerful touch, saying, "I love to pray and hold their hands." For some, the touch *was* the prayer (Martin) or was spiritual in and of itself: "Human touch is, I feel, it's spiritual" (Mona). Jane said, "I lay my hand on her head – so very conscious of the sacred power of touch in prayer. It connects in ways we cannot explain." Amelio provided a theological grounding for touch during prayer, specifically within the healthcare context: "Even Jesus used symbols when he was healing or laying on hands, touching the sick person. That's why we lay hands and we pray meditatively." These moments of touch were critical for the prayer practices themselves, but also for the social relations evident in the tactile prayers in healthcare. From the perspective of many of our participants, healthcare settings are spaces where social touch is quite limited and is much more clinical: "The touch in hospital is syringes, bed baths, pulling, pushing, often associated with pain" (Martin). By reaching out and holding a patient's or resident's hand, one provided for a physical need, and a different kind of touch experience: "A lot of people are isolated from any sort of physical touch in hospital, and so they like having their hand held" (Margaret). As such, the relationship between the person who was providing and the person who was receiving the prayerful touch was strengthened; the touch revealed "equality" and "respect" (Frida).

Prayerful touch also revealed transgression. Naomi, a healthcare professional, explained that with the increasing automation of healthcare, the use of technology to monitor and note patient charts, means that healthcare professionals can "see" patients without touching them. She explained that "when we talk about patients, not having or feeling the compassion or having compassionate care by nurses, it's because we don't touch them anymore. We're touching patients less and less." Nursing scholar Pam Smith (2012) suggests that a division between caring and technical nursing has become increasingly entrenched, and one of the clearest examples was that nurses were too wedded to routine to provide caring touch to their patients. Because of this routinized intention of touch in the healthcare setting, prayerful touch inevitably transgressed the norm.

Prayer and touch could also transgress healthcare norms concerned with "ethical, professional practice." Participants at several sites discussed the possible ethical issues that could arise with touching a resident or patient during prayer. Martin shared the ethics behind the question of touch: "What they write in the counsellor chaplain's handbook is that touch is a fundamental human gesture. It can communicate good and bad, so you must be careful.... My first ever week started with the question of the use of touch in the hospital setting. Absolutely the minimum and never with minors and never with people who are not capable of consent." Martin explained that while one must still be careful to work within these ethical boundaries, prayerful touch still pushed those boundaries, especially in moments near death. He elaborated, "With someone who's dying I can tell you that's the most reassuring thing you can ever do for someone," but Martin also made it clear that he always allows patients to take his hand, rather than imposing it on them. This careful navigation was essential, as one risks being "accused of harassment or touching" (Amelio). Taryn (chaplain) explained further the ethics around touch: "Touch is a big question. We don't want to impose touch on a patient. And yet for some patients it's significant and it's meaningful, so navigating that is always sensitive." While chaplains were careful in engaging in prayerful touch, many said it was an essential aspect of many prayer experiences in the healthcare setting.

Prayerful touch could also transgress socio-cultural norms and boundaries, especially if it was not part of one's familial, cultural, or religious life. Gender norms sometimes featured in how touch, prayer, and the healthcare context intersected. Mona shared how prayer and touch could transgress traditional gender lines in her role of chaplain:

> The men will ask you to pray for them and maybe touch them on their head, which I used to find strange in the beginning, because Muslim men, they're so conservative.... So when I'm in hospital, and I explain what I'm doing, because they think they want you to make this prayer for them, and in their culture, after you make the prayer, they want you to touch them ... so it doesn't matter for him when he is sick, if I was a man or if I was a woman but I'm doing the prayer and that's what he needs.... He probably wouldn't talk to me outside the hospital.

Although certain cultural and religious norms would dictate that these men could not have a non-family member of the opposite sex touch them, within this specific context (the healthcare context) and within this specific practice (prayer), these lines were sometimes crossed.

While outside hospital walls one may not engage in touch with people from different social or status groups, within hospital walls these social boundaries were traversed through prayerful touch. Lock (1993) suggests that research shows how "social categories are literally inscribed on and into the body, which ... acts as signifier of local social and moral worlds" (135). In the foundational work of anthropologist Mary Douglas (1966), social and cultural norms about cleanliness construct ideas about "otherness" such that one would not venture to physically touch someone who is perceived as "dirty" or "dangerous." These boundaries can, however, be reinforced in healthcare contexts, through professional norms of hygiene, which in turn portray meanings about acceptance, worth, and status. Martin further said, "It's the most awful experience of my life in this setting where I'd gone to see a patient, I'd shaken hands with the patient, and before meeting the next patient, you wash your hands to move on. But ... before going to the next patient, the one I'd just seen, saw me washing my hands ... and that was horrendous because that patient may have got completely the wrong understanding." Taryn described a situation where she engaged in prayerful touch with a patient who was viewed as "dirty, and unkempt, and tough on the team, and an addict." She explained how in this prayer experience the woman grabbed her hand and began praying for her: "This woman who wouldn't be the average person that I would run into in a church environment ... I was moved by the authenticity of the whole experience and humbled by it, thinking, 'My God, you're so in this space.'" Moreover, "the senses do not always work together or convey the same message;" what anthropologists Sarah Pink and David Howes call "sensory dissonance" (Pink and Howes 2010, 335). It is only through an anthropology of the senses, through taking the sense experience in all aspects seriously, that one gets the whole picture. Like Pink and Howes's statement about the "holy man who looks ugly but emits a fragrant odour of sanctity" (335), the experience of prayerful touch that Taryn had with this patient transgressed the boundaries and norms that the sense of sight put in place. Prayerful touch, then, transgressed the boundary between transcendence and imminence; it made the transcendental sensible (Meyer 2006).

The sensory experience of prayer went beyond the traditional five senses to include a "sixth sense" of intuition, when senses and emotions worked together to affect occurrences of prayer. Chaplains in London and Vancouver used their whole body to read prayer situations with patients. Andreas explained this prayerful intuiting: "I have this feeling and I go to the ward, and I walk into a room, and I see this patient sobbing. Nobody has seen her sobbing, nobody has seen her distressed, and I get to the bedside and I tell her who I am, and then she tells me what happened to her. And I feel like, who guided me there? Which is exactly what they needed, so it's sometimes by a rational approach; we do all these assessments, referrals, but other times we do work intuitively. Because we have to use our intuitive minds, healing requires intuition as well. It's not always an instrumental process." During a walking interview, Margaret also said, "There's no hard and fast rule as to when you come across either the opportunity or the need or the willingness to pray and I think it requires intuition." One must be able to read the emotions and sensorial factors and feel out the appropriate and timely prayer response. Yet sometimes this intuition is not so straightforward, as Zara suggested: "I'm surprised when people request prayer, so I don't always get it. I value that intuitive sense, but it's not always there." These examples revealed the intersubjective nature of emotion as written about by sociologists Ole Riis and Linda Woodhead (2010, 27): "the reflective flow of individual emotionality from one person to another and back again." Intuition, and moments of prayer that were perceived through the bodily, sensorial, and emotional experiences in the hospital came about not only through "mysterious intuition" but were also fostered through a "developed mutual awareness, and skilled interpretation of one another's thoughts, actions, speech, tone, movements and gestures" (27).

Throughout this chapter we have shown how material objects and bodies made the sacred real and present, allowing individuals to transgress boundaries and norms in healthcare settings in unexpected ways. Knitted within participants' narratives of prayer, materiality contributed to a greater understanding of lived religion (McGuire 2008). Because of the healthcare settings, which often privilege certain types of care over others, patients might have to adjust their embodied spiritual, religious, and prayer practices. The question then became how to accommodate embodied practice when patients, residents, staff, and others could not follow certain rules or desires. That is, when faced with material, embodied, and sensorial obstacles to prayer in the healthcare setting, what did people do? Sociologist Meredith McGuire (2008) suggests that historically, when people think about religion and spirituality, they think about a certain set of practices and beliefs created and enforced by specific institutions or institutional structures. However, she argues that when looking at people's everyday, lived experience, we see that religion and spirituality are multifaceted, diverse, and malleable. She states, "At the level of the individual, religion is not fixed, unitary, or even coherent" (12). In our study we observed that on the individual, lived level, people adjusted and adapted to move with and beyond the material and the sensorial to engage their prayer practices. This revealed how prayer could transgress ideas and norms about "medical bodies," and when, how, and who could perform prayer in the clinical setting. We continue this discussion of how the material, both created and natural, could affect lived experiences of prayer via the arts and nature in the next chapter.

Arts and Nature
in Lived Experiences of Prayer

Sonya Sharma and Melania Calestani

A field note: With other children and adults, I too stop to stare at the beauty and languid swimming of the colourful fish. The popular aquarium is an example of the porosity of nature and art. Slowing down to look is like stopping to look at a painting – a visual feast for the eyes. This interruption is welcomed after the hectic pace of travel to the site. Watching the fish seems like leisure time, transgressing my busy day and the clinical space and priorities surrounding me.

London is a city historically known for its opportunities to participate in and experience the arts, whether at national galleries and theatres, dance, music and opera houses, cinemas, or local endeavours that include community choirs, amateur drama companies, and arts and crafts groups and festivals. While London has well-known parks, canals, and the river Thames, it is London's landmarks such as London Bridge, Westminster Abbey, St. Paul's Cathedral, and Piccadilly Circus that are often prominent and featured in pieces of art (e.g., Claude Monet, L.S. Lowry, or Joseph Mallord William Turner). Many come to the city to see the historical architecture and to experience the diverse range of the arts, from plays by William Shakespeare to musicals *The Lion King* and *The Book of Mormon* to the Tate Modern art gallery. Several places of worship, both religious and secular, uphold the arts and cultivate them as a way to draw people into experiences of wonder or the sacred (e.g., the Sunday Assembly at Conway Hall or St. Martin-in-the-Fields Anglican Church).

In contrast, Vancouver is a city known for its mountains, oceans, lakes, and parks. Many in the city have easy access to walks along the beach, hikes in the forest, and exercise and leisure activities in "green and blue spaces" (Finlay et al. 2015). Vancouver has its own history with the arts, one in which nature features prominently. Emily Carr's paintings depict the beauty and wildness of British Columbian rain forests. Indigenous artists have conveyed their long history and relationship to the animals and the land (e.g., Bill Reid and Lawrence Paul Yuxweluptun). Even contemporary photographer Jeff Wall (1990) has captured mundane Vancouver suburbs against the backdrop of the North Shore Mountains. As noted in other chapters, Vancouver, located in the Pacific Northwest, "has natural amenities that can be considered as a resource for spirituality that has the power to satisfy some people's need for inspiration, awe, and divine connection" (Ferguson and Tamburello 2015, 298).

London and Vancouver offer different opportunities to engage in arts and nature, and these in turn mediate prayer in varied ways, just as the materiality of the body and objects were shown to do in the previous chapter. Arts and nature are dealt with together in this chapter because of how they alter and transgress experiences of clinical contexts and temporalities. First, we briefly discuss what is meant by the arts and nature and how they have been incorporated into healthcare. Second, we describe the presence of the arts and nature at our research sites in London and Vancouver. Third, we move on to participants' accounts of arts and nature in their experiences of prayer, considering them in clinical settings and temporalities. We conclude by discussing how the intertwinement of the arts, nature, and prayer could both reinforce and challenge inequalities felt among religious and non-religious groups.

ARTS AND NATURE IN HEALTHCARE

At our research sites there was a plethora of the arts on offer, which included fine arts (i.e., architecture, graphics, painting, and sculpture) and performing arts (i.e., dance, drama, and music) and "contemporary arts practices" such as arts, crafts, and music sessions. *Contemporary arts practices* "is an umbrella term for describing arts practice in relation to society through various modes [such as] through elective practice, self-organized activities, documentaries, trans-disciplinary research practices and participatory and socially engaged art" (Broderick 2011, 102). These kinds of arts practices are particularly attuned to engaging with the social and burgeoned from the 1990s onward (Bishop 2005; Staricoff and Clift 2011). In the United States, the Society for the Arts in Healthcare was formed in 1991 and more recently transformed to call itself the Arts & Health Alliance. In Canada, there is the Arts and Health Network, founded in 2005, which includes Arts Health BC, a community and founding member of the larger Canadian network. The Arts and Health Forum in London formed in 2008 and is part of the wider National Alliance for Arts, Health & Wellbeing that launched in 2012. Key aims of these organizations are to articulate and promote the relationship between arts and health and the impact creativity can have on engagement, coping, and increasing qualities of good health. "Arts programs within healthcare have become increasingly mainstreamed and expected" (Lambert 2015, xv). The presence of arts practices in healthcare has grown, and research in this area has increased with investigations of how the arts in healthcare contribute to patient and staff wellbeing (e.g., All-Parliamentary Group 2017; Broderick 2011; Fleischer and Grehan 2016; Wilson et al. 2016).

Like the arts, nature in healthcare has faced a similar trajectory and can be defined in many ways and encompass many things and experiences. Nature includes the "nonhuman, living flora and fauna, running water, air and weather, geological landscapes and processes, and nature in the built environment such as parks, community gardens and allotments, street trees and indoor plants" (Hartig et al. 2014, 208). People may also experience nature from inside a "building or vehicle, when viewing photographs or films or within virtual reality set-ups" (208). Psychologists Rachel Kaplan and Stephen Kaplan (1989) noted nature's many aspects and its significance to people's experiences of home, work, and life, from the ordinary exposure of it through an office, home, or hospital window, to actively being in it – whether hiking, swimming, walking – and its effects on health. Since their work, numerous studies have examined the link between nature and health (e.g., Maller et al. 2006; Mitchell 2013; Nilsson, Sangster, and Konijnendijk 2011; Pretty 2004). More recently, the role of nature in healthcare has also been considered. Many hospitals have constructed gardens on hospital grounds or within the hospitals themselves, where patients, families, and staff can sit among a variety of plants, flowers, waterfalls, fountains, butterflies, or aquariums. Given these spaces, studies have been conducted to assess their impact on health and well-being, noting their capacity to promote healing, happiness, and relaxation (e.g., van der Riet et al. 2017). Others have studied hospital architecture and environments and found that access to daylight and fresh air can be crucial to positive impacts on experiences of healthcare (e.g., van den Berg 2005).

Research on both the arts and nature in healthcare is diverse, with scholars approaching the study of them in different ways, whether qualitatively or quantitatively. A challenge for instituting more arts and nature within healthcare is how they conform to evidence-based models of evaluation that seek to demonstrate positive clinical outcomes for patients. In this chapter, we do not posit the arts and nature in service of clinical health benefits but interrogate how they could generate and be part of lived experiences of prayer among participants. But first, a brief description of the ways art and nature were present in the contexts we conducted our research.

THE PRESENCE OF THE ARTS AND NATURE
AT OUR RESEARCH SITES

At a London site, a fundraising body was tasked to support the arts' ability to transform the clinical experience and environment for patients, families, and staff. This included bringing together artists and designers to think about how, for example, light and sound could affect the patient and clinical experience of waiting for and receiving treatment. There were participatory arts for older people who had suffered a stroke or who had dementia. Arts, crafts, and music sessions took place along with dance and movement classes. Performances of music and dance and by theatre groups aimed to improve the hospital experience for all. One of the first things each of us noticed when we visited these sites was the art that graced the walls that included digital and visual art. At our research sites in London and Vancouver, art was also present in the designated sacred spaces, such as fine art, religious icons and artifacts, and specially gifted carpets to a Muslim prayer room and one First Nations sacred space, which was circular and patterned with Indigenous imagery.

At a Vancouver site, the arts were also supported by a fundraising body. However, the presence of the arts differed. Often one could view religious iconography, abstract generic art, nature photography, and sculptures of crosses. Indigenous art was also prominent. These seemed to be part of the clinical setting's decor, not necessarily a promoted feature like in London. In Vancouver, some artistic endeavours were characterized as "happy kitsch" by the research team. At one healthcare setting, fake leis of neon pink and orange flowers bordered the windows of a nursing station. Some of our Vancouver sites also offered arts, crafts, and music sessions. On one visit we witnessed a man playing guitar encouraging an organized sing-along to those seated around him. Staff and patients appreciated the sense of well-being that the arts could bring, but they were cultivated differently than in London. As explained above, this is partly due to the city of London itself, a leading city for the arts, and the funding and support the London sites received.

In Vancouver, healthcare spaces were not far from high-end shops, hotels, concert halls and cinemas, and places for religious worship. Most obvious, though, was their proximity to nature, such as the ocean, forest, and local parks with benches to sit, relax, and eat one's lunch. From several sites you could view the mountains, the river, or the ocean. The naturistic views could themselves be considered the art of nature and reprieve from suffering within clinical spaces. Where the arts could be viewed at our London sites, in Vancouver it was the beautiful vistas and views, the art of nature on display. Nature was never far from our research sites in Vancouver. At one of the long-term care facilities, they had recently renovated an outdoor seating area where one could hear the sounds of waterfalls or sit among potted plants and flowers. This area overlooked a green lawn and trees that surrounded the building. In London, nature could be found via inner and outer gardens, and not too far away via parks, a cemetery, and the river Thames. Many would argue that "in reality nature is all around us. Whether we live in densely packed cities or rural countryside, we are part of a complex ecosystem with the plants, animals, land, air and water that surround us" (Wellcome Trust 2017, n.p.). In contrast to London, though, our Vancouver sites had nature right on their doorstep. The ability to be in nature was for many much more accessible, just as the arts were for many in London. In the next sections, we focus on participants' accounts of art and nature in lived experiences of prayer, beginning with the ways that arts, nature, and prayer could transgress clinical settings.

TRANSGRESSING CLINICAL CONTEXTS
AND TEMPORALITIES

Clinical Contexts

Some of our participants in London and Vancouver perceived health-care settings as being too "secular." When defining this term, they talked about the difficulty to pray in a clinical context that was not conducive "to feeling particularly alive spiritually," as Kirstie (citizen) told us in London. Andreas, a chaplain in Vancouver, explained that "secular" in this context implied a separation between the body and the soul, and a lack of connection between the two. He went on to explain that the clinical context was experienced as not inclusive enough of all the spiritual needs of patients. The intertwinement of arts, nature, and prayer could therefore transgress the clinical experience, altering it for some of our participants.

Theologian James McCullough (2015) articulates the relationship between the arts and spirituality in terms of aesthesis (sensory perception) and ascesis (disciplined spiritual activity), mediated and facilitated by the arts. The arts can be a catalyst for deep meaning, reflection, and prayer in healthcare settings, but for some of our participants the arts were prayer itself. For instance Chiara, a non-religious citizen in London, said, "For me [prayer] means dancing, which is great. I think a prayer can be in so many different ways. What is a prayer? It's an externalization of a feeling and a request. Prayer is normally a request or an act of communication." Performing arts were described as creating an ambience or a vehicle that could nurture or manifest prayer and spirituality and reflect the spirit of the person. Maryanne, an administrator in Vancouver, said, "Those who are musicians, giving them a space to play the guitar or providing art supplies to clients who are really artistic and creative and then letting them show that, to me comprises of looking after the spirit of who they are." Dancing, music, singing (e.g., Christmas carols) and embodied movement in general were described as instrumental for facilitating spirituality and prayer. For instance, Rinaldo, a chaplain in Vancouver, told us, "I enjoy going to Mass and of course there [the beauty of the arts] is more formal. Then as I'm walking, I'll say the rosary or the Divine Mercy or when the weather's good and you see the blue sky, I say a thank you to God." Rinaldo made clear references to how the surrounding environment could trigger moments of prayer, the inspiration provided by artistic beauty in a service or in nature.

The impact of the performing arts on their audiences was also apparent. As researchers we observed some of the performances that took place at one of our London sites. When doing so, the attention shifted from the embodiment of prayer expressed by performers, like in the case of Chiara, to the impact that it might have on the audience's experiences of spirituality and/or prayer. One week we sat and watched Indian classical dancing. On that day, the music filled the air of the hospital, and it felt as if the audience was transported to a different country. Visitors, in-patients, outpatients, and staff members all stopped to observe the two dancers, who were thanking Mother Earth and moving in their colourful dresses. Anthropologists Simon Coleman and John Elsner's work on creativity and spirituality explicates (1998) that aesthetic ideas can serve as bridges to spiritual categories, releasing transcendent senses and emotions in a (medical) context that is often assumed to be unemotional and cold. The performing arts could transgress the clinical nature of hospitals.

Similarly, in Vancouver, our participants talked about the inspiration they took from the outside landscape, characterized by the scenic mountain range and the ocean on the horizon, and the community gardens. Importantly, religious studies scholar Paul Bramadat describes the kind of experiences people can have in nature, particularly in the Pacific Northwest, as "reverential naturalism": "The sense that being out in nature is not just a place where one does spirituality or religion, but it is a medium through which it is done ... one is reconfigured, transformed and transfixed by that experience" (Bramadat 2018). Jane, a chaplain, told us that "nature can help facilitate prayer because one would be hard pressed to find someone who doesn't like nature." She added that getting outside provides a feeling of "freedom." Walter, another chaplain, reflected on the relationship of natural beauty to the sacred and why he used in particular the space of nature to pray with patients: "It's nature. It's beauty. The way I've described nature is that nature takes you outside of yourself. It points to a creator. I think it gets people into that transcendent realm. It draws you to something beyond yourself, a life force that can create this kind of beauty." In London, for some participants, nature provided a form of connection external to oneself. George (administrator) said, "I feel that if I am in an environment, a rural countryside, then I feel very much [a connection outside of myself]." Similarly, Franco, a citizen we interviewed, described his "greatest connection is with the spiritual in nature." He told us about a favourite woodland "where it's very quiet and people can connect with loved ones they've lost and find they haven't really lost them at all.... Out there it is like a cathedral with the branches of the trees and wonderful to connect there with infinite spirit, with God." In our study and others, many people discuss how spirituality can be achieved or felt when they are in contact or in harmony with the non-human environment (Thin 2009, 31), feeling at peace when surrounded by nature.

Gardens were identified as meaningful bridges to spiritual categories and the healthcare contexts, in which we carried out research, designed specific spaces to put people in contact with nature (see, for example figure 9.1). Sometimes they even brought nature into these settings via digital landscape art. For instance, at one London site, a large-scale image of a coastal village had embedded digital effects whereby the water was rippling. Luis (chaplain) mentioned that the garden in the hospital in which he worked was inextricably linked with his spiritual background:

> We associate so much being in touch with nature to get good spirit and release bad spirits ... vibes. We believe that the earth and the soil and the ground, the plants will take our bad energy and then we will get good energy from them [plants]. It's like carbon dioxide and oxygen.... I believe that some of the energy taken during the interaction with patients, unconsciously you are receiving some of this energy, good or bad and you are giving also. Every person I encounter, I talk with, there's always an exchange of energy. [Human beings] exchange energy and I come here [to the garden] to unload this bad energy.

From these comments, we saw that gardens and nature were important not only in the healing of patients, but also for staff members' well-being. Gardens served as meaningful metaphors to talk about the social relations of prayer in healthcare settings. Moments of prayer were conceived as exchanges of energy and the gardens as a means to find harmony again, showing how engaging in prayer and spiritual care with patients could at times feel like an emotional burden (Reimer-Kirkham and Sharma et al. 2018) that required "unloading" through therapeutic spaces such as healing gardens.

Through these different examples, gardens and nature could enable belonging among multi-faith users of the hospital, catering to different needs and offering a mediating role for different individuals,

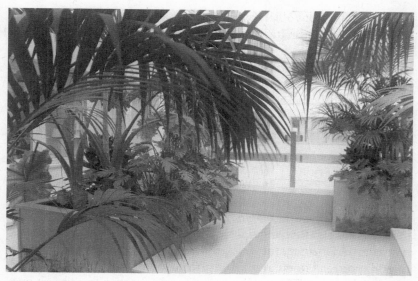

9.1 Indoor garden

despite their religious or non-religious affiliation. George elaborated
on the importance of a garden in the context of healthcare: "It's an
important place. I consider it as being like the other religious spaces.
It's a refuge. I think, even with spiritual care team members, it's considered to be an important space. Even for the patients and families
that don't have a religious affiliation … it can be a quiet place where
they can go for some quiet time." Through our data, we observed that
nature and the arts had a mediating role that helped to transgress clinical contexts in powerful and subjective ways, especially when some
felt that hospital contexts were "too secular." Linda Woodhead (2017)
writes about "no religion" as a category similar to "religious" and discusses through her work the rising number of nones in the UK. A
question then arises regarding how hospitals can become inclusive of
all the different religious and non-religious needs and definitions of
care. As highlighted by anthropologist Elana Buch (2015, 279), *care* in
English-speaking places connotes both affective concern (caring
about) and practical action (caring for); often this duality of meaning
contributes to beliefs that caring actions are best or most naturally
motivated by caring feelings (see also Tronto 1994; and Ungerson
1990). However, the pressure of the clinical context linked with the
acuity of patients may not always allow for the affective concern and

the practical action to be linked together. As observed, arts and nature were one way in which hospital staff and users made this link.

Clinical Temporalities

Clinical environments such as hospitals are shaped by time: the urgency of providing treatment, the scheduled times of giving medicine, the routines of care given by healthcare professionals, the time needed to rest and repair the body. But what happens when the intersection of art, nature, and prayer transgress these temporalities? What impact do they have on the busy life of hospitals? Historian of religion Mircea Eliade ([1959] 1987) thought of time in two ways: sacred time and profane time. The former is when one views oneself as involved in "a primordial mythical time made present" (68). The latter focuses on the experience of everyday activities. By marking these two times, they are not the same but different (Kirk 1990). Time taken to be with a higher power such as in church or in nature can be qualitatively different from other ordinary mundane times (Kirk 1990, 10). Paul, a chaplain, reflected on the art found in the chapel of one London site. He explained his process of accessing his relationship to the divine amidst a high-paced ethos of care:

> At that hospital, there is something there for me, which represents my belief in the way I want to express it; for example, the painting, whether you have any faith or not, or whether you believe in the resurrection or not, the simple fact that it's there, actually you are looking at something that challenges something in here [*points to self*] and even though you might be looking at something of a faith belief, it's a painting that is expressing something, or at least it's challenging the mind, while behind you there's a whole hospital going on. Sometimes people go there to get away from whatever is going on.... At that hospital the calmness is created by some of the imaginary.

In this excerpt, Paul described a "calmness" and time away and apart from the "whole hospital that is going on" around him. The art provided a vehicle for which to engage with the divine imaginary and to mark a sacred time and space. The chapel became a sanctuary or a refuge amidst a hectic hospital and city. Collins and colleagues (2007, 121) learned that some chaplains regarded sacred spaces as "defensible spaces" that are distinct and necessary for staff, families, and patients to feel safe and quiet. Andreas discussed the importance of architectural design to one's relationship to something God-like: "You go into a big space like a cathedral. And there was a reason that it was so large, to feel this magnificent presence of something." Similarly chapel spaces within healthcare settings are often set apart and are typically quiet and peaceful where one can sit, reflect, pray, and spend time.

As with designated sacred spaces such as chapels, gardens as informal sacred spaces could also interrupt clinical temporalities with a sense of sacred time. Luis reflected on his use of the garden at a London site: "[Nature is important,] especially for other faiths because they might be able to connect with God our Creator through the beauty of nature, especially Buddhists and Hindus. Some Sikh doctors or nurses may come here. Sometimes I come here when I'm tired and I need some quiet time. I sit down here. It's often on my way to somewhere else. I go around the wards for one hour or one hour and half and then I stay here." Some of our London participants talked about this garden extensively, despite their religious and non-religious affiliations. Tall potted plants surrounded benches, and many staff members went there for serenity and renewal. Not unlike the chapel, it was set apart, away from other bustling areas of the hospital and the dark corridors of the wards. At a Vancouver site there was an outdoor terraced garden. In what was technically a smoke-free space, it was not unusual to see staff and patients there have a cigarette, to take a break from time spent on the ward. Jane described this space to us: "I brought you out to the smoking area in the garden. I see people out there and they're on their own and stuff is going through their heads when they're out there. They're going through something when they're out there. To my mind that's almost like a place of prayer." These descriptions suggested that a separation between sacred and profane times and spaces were not so clearly demarcated. They appeared to be fluid, a part of each other, where the mundane meets the otherworldly, where the profane becomes sacred. Sociologist Emile Durkheim ([1915] 2008) suggests that the sacred and the profane are mutually exclusive, yet he also contends that the boundaries between sacred and profane can be trespassed. It is further argued by sociologist Nicholas Demerath III (2007, 66) that "sacralization is the process by which the secular becomes sacred or other new forms of the sacred emerge, whether in matters of personal faith or institutional practice." In the moments where chaplains visited the gardens or used the cigarette break to create sacred moments and spaces that were transcendent and set apart, the possibility for prayer could occur.

Thus, being able to create or view art works, be mindful about them, use them as a source of healing, meditation and prayer while receiving or waiting for treatment seeped into clinical timelines. Kirstie, who had grown up in London and had spent time at one of the London sites, spoke about the artwork: "I find the artwork in the hospital quite enjoyable, even uplifting, when I go there for out-patient appointments." Elaine, an administrator at a London site, described prayer as "reflection" and expressed similar sentiments about the artwork: "When you walk around the hospital, you see a lot of both staff and patients looking at the artwork and talking about it, and you see the children pointing at an indoor sculpture, and if you took the aquarium actually as an artwork ... But on a personal basis one of the reasons that I like to come to work here is that you can go around the corner and see another piece of art. It lifts the spirit." Kirstie and Elaine connected to the artwork within the time of waiting and amid the workday of walking around the hospital. The time they took to view the art might be thought of in linear terms with a beginning and an end. However, the connection they had to the artwork "lifted their spirits." The sacred merged into the ordinary activities of an appointment and the going to and from an office. Sacred and profane temporalities transgressed each other. Kirk describes "what happens in the course of this journeying is that 'time for God' moves from a selected time to 'all the time'" (1990, 13). Time for God or prayer can be planned and set apart and also unplanned and all the time, when temporalities of prayer in relation to art and nature are non-linear and are time spent within time, blurring temporalities of clinical routines and prayer. Demerath III (2000, 4) states, "Too often we look for the sacred under a religious street lamp, when we should be searching amongst other experiences in the middle of the block." Like Kirstie and Elaine's experiences pointed to, the sacred was found in other situations, times, and spaces external to formally religious spaces (Bramadat 2018; Kong 2010). These were just as important and could, moreover, highlight inequalities felt by religious and non-religious groups and individuals – issues we explore in the concluding section of this chapter.

ARTS AND NATURE IN PRAYER:
REINFORCING AND CHALLENGING INEQUALITIES

For the most part, we have written about positive examples of arts and nature in the lived experiences of prayer and how they positively transgressed clinical contexts and temporalities. Paradoxically, the presence of art could highlight inequalities between groups, potentially limiting possibilities for prayer. For example, a Muslim administrator at one of our Vancouver sites stated that it was difficult for her to say prayers at work, in part because of the busyness of the setting, but more because it was difficult to find space conducive to prayers. Of the chapel on site, she said, "There is too much happening in there for me to be able to settle down for prayer." In this participant's opinion, the religious iconography representing a tradition other than her own made it difficult for her to pray. Her comment raised the question of the accessibility of art, and who has aesthetic spaces available to them for prayer. How do the arts and nature by way of prayer reinforce and challenge social and religious inequalities?

In London and Vancouver, where both fine and performing art could be experienced in the public areas of healthcare spaces, the clinical areas could be different, without pieces of art, leaving us wondering how the art upon entry could be evenly spread to other areas. Towards the end of our research, there was more effort and plans by the healthcare sites to put visual and digital art onto wards, lounges, and quiet spaces. In addition, during our time visiting the sites in London and Vancouver, much of the fine art on display was abstract – a form that has been criticized as elitist; is it a postmodern look into meaninglessness or a conversation piece (Meecham and Sheldon 2013)? Historically in the West in the early twentieth century, "art appreciation was seen as both reactionary and elitist, a powerful representative of class values" and "connoisseurship supported by notions about aesthetics acted as criteria about what constituted good taste" (xx). Particular forms of art and knowledge have thus been associated with particular Western values and class norms, which can result in the exclusion of a range of individuals and groups (Bourdieu 1984). Arts and nature were generally received as a positive aspect of healthcare contexts, and while approaches to art have evolved and the arts as a whole have become more inclusive, modern art and its histories were still present. Connor, an administrator at one of our London sites, described how the art that one saw upon entering one health-care setting created good feelings about working in that space, and yet simultaneously had the capacity to conceal structural inequalities among staff and users. Although much art was abstract, there was some evidence of opening to more diversity in the art portrayed. At one site some art depicted Islam and Muslim ethnicity. In the West itself there have been racialized discourses of religion surrounding Muslim groups because of the 2001 bombings in New York and sub-sequent terrorist attacks in London in 2007, and other European cities. But the hospital's values are to be open and respectful of all, and the presence of this art and art that also depicted Christian symbols (see chapter 8) and Indigenous imagery (see chapter 3) could create a sense of well-being, belonging, acknowledging faith traditions and spiritual practices.

In contrast, nature in facilitating prayer could be thought of as not reinforcing inequalities. It is assumed that everyone has some experi-ence of or access to nature, whether through domestic plant life, pic-tures of it, parks and trees in hospital neighbourhoods, or views of it from hospital windows. However, inequalities could be observed in access to garden spaces within and proximate to healthcare settings. Some patients were without the help and luxury of a bed next to a window or of being wheeled outside or to an indoor garden. For those who took a non-religious stance, with art or nature potentially informing their non-religious practices (e.g., Humanist, spiritual, Pagan, none), a lack of access to time and space could be felt as deeply unequal. It was important for some of the non-religious we inter-viewed to have access to time for reflection and spaces of beauty and solace. Naomi, a healthcare professional who identified as non-religious, explained "If you were religious and need to pray, what does that mean for those who don't? I think there can be an imbalance, where we're giving and allowing time for some and not for others who don't have a faith or want to do that. For me, that creates inequality." Stanley, an administrator and also non-religious, said, "We need to spend time thinking about the environment being beautiful and restful and conducive to recovery, mindfulness, meditation. These are spaces that if you're not overtly religious, give you that same kind of solace.... And yet for a largely secular society, healthy or ill, little thought is given to that." Issues of time within healthcare set-tings, and a lack of access to spaces that were made pleasing and peaceful by the presence or not of art and nature, could therefore reinforce inequalities felt among both religious and non-religious groups, limiting expressions of prayer. Some of our chaplains asked, "How do we provide for the non-religious?" This is becoming a more pressing concern, given their rise in number in both cities. Perhaps Naomi's and Stanley's reflections on time and space point to where to begin.

The presence of arts and nature via formal and informal religious and non-religious spaces and practices could simultaneously challenge inequalities too. Healthcare settings are public spaces (see chapter 2) and are frequently used by community constituents for their cafés, canteens, conference rooms, gardens, and designated religious spaces. Chapels and multi-faith spaces are often a part of corporate identities of hospitals because of the prominent place of art that can consist within them. Art can draw people to these spaces, bringing attention to the significance of spiritual care and to the importance of beauty to prayer, health, and well-being. For many, it might be their first exposure to different art forms and internationally renowned artists, who performed at or were displayed on hospital walls in both London and Vancouver. It could also be someone's first experience of gardening, whereby one of our research sites had a community garden that grew vegetables and flowers. Healthcare settings can open up other kinds of opportunities for healing, growth, and development. It can also be argued that when people have access to the arts and to nature it increases their knowledge and exposure to the social and cultural life around them. In his research on social class, sociologist Mike Savage (2015) highlights that engaging with publicly supported cultural facilities and activities contributes to the development of artistic and cultural knowledges. In London and Vancouver, cities of deprivation and prosperity, there are numerous public spaces and facilities to engage with the arts and nature, from parks and streetscapes to libraries, schools, and community centres (Stevenson and Magee 2017). Healthcare settings are part of this landscape too.

The intersection of arts, nature, and prayer in our research sites uncovered the fact that clinical settings and temporalities were not always distinctly biomedical. These contexts were transgressed by arts, nature, and prayer. Also, if prayer is a lens onto religion in the public sphere, its convergence with the arts and nature revealed visible and invisible inequalities marked and felt among those religious and non-religious. And yet the transgressions of art, nature, and prayer in the public space of healthcare demonstrated a capacity to move toward encounter, meaningfulness, relief of suffering, and belonging amongst individuals and groups, opening up spaces where equality could be experienced and nurtured for all.

CONCLUSION

The Power of Prayer

Sonya Sharma and Sheryl Reimer-Kirkham

In early spring 2018 an exhibition entitled *Living with Gods: Peoples, Places and Worlds Beyond* was held at the British Museum in London. Focusing on numerous objects from their collection, the exhibition attended to how people believe versus what they believe. Historical artifacts from the Ice Age to current everyday objects were on display, including those used for prayer. They conveyed how practices of prayer have long been with us, helping people make sense of their lives and the unknown; generate meaning, order, and understanding; and engender connection between people and other-worldly beings. The objects of prayer on display in the British Museum, however, also illustrated the importance of interrogating historical and geographical contexts and structures of power (i.e., colonialism and patriarchy) in the understanding of religious practices. The power of prayer stems not only from its mystical and metaphysical qualities, but also the historical and social structures within which it is situated and practised. Such social relations of prayer were at the heart of our analysis in this study. In this concluding chapter we begin with summarizing key themes of the book by applying the metaphor of curtains to our synopsis of the chapters. We then explore what the study of prayer in city healthcare settings reveals about religion in the public sphere, what it opens us up to, and what it points us toward.

CURTAINS AS A METAPHOR FOR UNDERSTANDING PRAYER IN HEALTHCARE SETTINGS

Stepping back to summarize the book, we were struck by how evocative curtains were in our data, helping us to interpret prayer in clinical contexts with added clarity, coherence, and depth. Curtains are a ubiquitous material object in healthcare settings. They can facilitate privacy and potentially heighten invisibility. They can create intimacy and distance between staff, patients, and families, and provide dignity for those suffering. Curtains can be perceived as a clear boundary between medical and non-medical procedures, but they are in fact porous, as other ways of the world peek in and seep through, including sound. For example, patients and staff overheard prayers being performed through curtained-off bedsides, resulting in them joining in or requesting prayers too. "Sometimes, the staff may come later and say, 'I am sorry, but I heard you behind the curtain. Could you pray with me?'" (Frances, chaplain, Vancouver). Despite curtains on the wards acting as a boundary for privacy, the act of prayer caused aspects of the private and public to blur. In the face of vulnerability, prayer was an intimate, public, and sometimes communal experience. As put by Mona, "It depends, sometimes you close the curtain, sometimes you don't. I've been praying with someone and somebody next door was repeating the prayer as well. They were Muslim, and I didn't have them on my list. When I finished, I went over to pray with them too.... The curtain doesn't make much difference, I think" (chaplain, London). Alluded to in this observation, and explicated in chapter 1, was the wide range of meanings and expressions of prayer in healthcare that evidenced social processes of revealing and concealing, blurring and crossing, connecting and distancing.

Such social processes were picked up in chapter 2. The implications of religious diversity played out on hospital wards, whereby participants made space for others' differences, including faith practices. Healthcare settings are complex social systems and microcosms of broader society where agreement, ambivalence, and conflict coincide. They are also where religions "cross and dwell" (Tweed 2006) and evidence that "religion is a persistent paradox" (Davie 2015), both growing and declining, not neutral and contributing to tension, solidarity, and equality. Staff and patients navigated living with diversity, and prayer was a way to respect common ground or keep respectful distance. Jane (chaplain, Vancouver) described this dynamic: "I was very conscious that we were on an open ward of four people. The patient in the bed directly next to hers was sitting up alert, only a thin curtain dividing us, as we shared prayer together."

In clinical contexts, making space for all (the theme of chapter 3) was not necessarily easy. A chaplain explained about the multi-faith space when two groups were using the space at the same time: "The curtains are not enough. Things were eventually worked out, but not without some conflict." Curtains erected in this space aimed to give different faith groups their area to pray and worship, but sounds, noise, and people entering or leaving the space could be disruptive, leading to conflict. These were in the end worked through, but such moments of worship and prayer amplified how geographies of prayer, formal and informal, were not static but constructed in the social relations between people. Curtains in the designated multi-faith space could denote formal spaces of prayer, while curtains on the wards could indicate informal spaces of prayer. Whether open or not, the porosity of bedside curtains resulted in unexpected moments and sites of prayer, exposing the malleability between sacred and profane and the fluidity of spaces.

The presence of curtains was symbolic of upholding hospital values and mission statements that included dignity and compassion towards patients and families. As presented in chapter 4, prayer showed up despite and because of organizational practices, policies, and values. The organizations signalled the value they placed on respect for spiritualities and religions through the designation of sacred spaces and resourcing of chaplaincy services. Curtains could be considered a metaphor for how organizational practices disclosed or foreclosed prayer, such as when organizations were not clear about their policies or did not resource chaplaincy services according to the clientele they served. Moreover, healthcare institutions could harbour hesitancies and ambivalences toward religions and spiritualities in part because of religious illiteracy amongst staff, but also because of clinical and social discourses that deem prayer and religion as irrelevant or as cultural difference of the Other.

In chapter 5 we focused our analysis on chaplains. Curtains were a way they navigated and respected the faith identities of patients, as indicated by Taryn: "It's my angst that drives me to ask, 'Would you like me to draw the curtain, would you like me to close the door?' 'No.' I've never had somebody say, 'Yes.' Never. I'm aware it is my piece" (chaplain, Vancouver). Chaplains, often the ones to pray for patients, families, and staff, took a patient-led or person-centred approach in order to assess the needs and circumstances of those receiving treatment and care. Heeding their needs was also in tandem with chaplains finding their way in healthcare contexts and among multidisciplinary teams and meetings. Prayer, when taken up by chaplains who were in liminal positions, was itself liminal in the clinical context. Chaplains operated along multiple axes of spiritual care, from religion-specific to generic, from team responsibility to specialist task, and from professionalism to advocacy. Prayer occurred across all of these dimensions, but models of chaplaincy, multi-faith and generic, while aimed to be inclusive, could also miss opportunities for prayer, with those unaffiliated or non-religious sometimes being overlooked.

The subject of chapter 6 was that prayer showed up behind the curtains of many clinical sites and wards. In efforts to offer spiritual care, prayer appeared not only for patients receiving palliative care, as often assumed, but was present in critical care, long-term care, and mental health and street clinics. It was present in the accompanying of patients in their final moments, during times of crisis, helping them to remember, affirming their personhood, and in countering social exclusion. Healthcare settings are contexts in which prayer becomes "de-localized," belonging to multiple spaces and participants discovering "contextual opportunities and constraints" in diverse clinical settings and within the wider social and physical formation of these spaces in cities (Hüwelmeier 2017).

Chapter 7 complicated common understandings of religious identities. While chaplains and other participants may have presented or been perceived to hold a particular religious identity, this did not mean they prayed only with those of their faith tradition. They prayed with many of different faiths, crossing boundaries of non-religious and religious traditions and identities. Yet, as Taryn suggested, closing the curtains was really about her comfort and ease, not the patient's. Should faith and indeed prayer be something the patient requested, religious identities could be amplified. As one chaplain said, "If you're absolutely certain of the person in the bed and their faith, then it's much easier. It's a real obstacle if you don't know, I think." Depending on who they found behind the curtain, such hesitancy and potential dilemmas confronted by participants demonstrated the tensions of moving between distinct (sui generis) and personal (lived religion) approaches to their own and others' faith identities, and modes of prayer. These were further entangled with intersectional approaches in that religious identities and the enactment of prayer were not separate from the structuring effects of gender, race, class, and sexuality.

Chapter 8 dealt with the materiality of prayer. Curtains were material objects that mediated prayer and the sacred. They could help to create a private space for people to tell their story, which led to or was interpreted as a prayer. Prayer was embodied, and bodies read prayer. As bodies leaned in or toward another to pray with or over, the senses aided in scanning and gleaning connection with the sacred. The senses could also limit and obstruct prayer because of bodily odours or bodily treatment and care. Also emotions were deeply embedded within the life of prayer. Many of our participants applied feeling words to describe meaningful moments of prayer. When chaplains took us on walking interviews, most often the spaces they took us to were where moments of prayer assisted in comforting panic, fear, or distress, or celebrating joy, relief, and recovery. Emotional geographies permeated the clinical settings because they were where people often felt a sense of emotional acuity or involvement (Davidson, Bondi, and Smith 2005), and hence they infused expressions and the materiality of prayer. Curtains were used to hide a dying or dead body, to separate life and death, symbolizing the liminal state between living and dying. Prayer and spiritual care were liminal and curtains emblematic, thus, of the social relations of prayer revealed in this study.

The role of arts and nature in relation to prayer were analyzed in chapter 9. Behind hospital curtains sometimes one found personal artifacts, such as photographs, religious icons, or prayer beads on bedside tables. Depending on where one was located, works of art were mounted on the walls so that patients and visitors had something pleasing to look at. Arts and nature had a way of coming through the curtains of "lifting the spirit." One chaplain told the story of a patient who heard opera music being sung in the hospital that she managed to hear from her bed. She said it got her through her hospitalization. Apart from potted plants, windows where one could view the sky, mountains, trees, or gardens outside made a difference, along with daylight. Whether inside or outside, gardens with big leafy palms or tall sunflowers could substitute for curtains to create a secluded alcove in which to have a quiet time or moment of prayer. Additionally, fine art that was resplendent and hung on the walls of our sites could veil lived inequalities among healthcare users. Likewise, they could expose and create a sense of belonging and healing among staff, residents, and patients. Art and nature as metaphors for curtains could be implicated in dynamics of equality and inequality, concealment and revelation.

In healthcare settings in Vancouver and London, prayer transgressed the boundaries of the sacred and the profane, the private and the public, the clinical and the non-clinical. Questioning prayer as transgression allowed us to understand how the sacred turns up, the constraints that prevent it, and the boundaries it crosses. Prayer as transgression queried "the moment where limits are transgressed, events happen, and rites are enacted where new social relations occur and we alter the 'once stable contours of institutions' and accelerate the process of change" (Hejduk 2010, 291). Prayer could disrupt the secular and rational order of healthcare contexts, to expose them as messy, complex, intimate, and unpredictable spaces where the mystical and transcendent erupted, percolated, and dwelled fleetingly and persistently. In this sense, prayer as transgression was transformative, even if it was sometimes viewed with suspicion or rejected by patients, residents, and staff. Transgression "pulled back the curtains" on prayer and, more broadly, religion in the public sphere of healthcare. In the last section we shift to ask what lessons can be derived and what new questions are posed, on account of pulling back these curtains. What does the study of prayer in healthcare in London and Vancouver reveal about religion in the public sphere? What does the study of prayer open us up to and point us toward?

WHAT DOES PRAYER IN HEALTHCARE SETTINGS REVEAL ABOUT RELIGION IN THE PUBLIC SPHERE?

Our intention with this project was not only to analyze expressions of prayer in healthcare settings, as interesting as this turned out to be, but also to view prayer as a window onto religion in the public sphere. In this section we focus on three contemporary developments made visible by this work: the pluralization, personalization, and politicization of prayer and religion.

Pluralization

In London and Vancouver, what does prayer in healthcare reveal about religion in the public sphere? Like the expressions of prayer we found in our study, the pluralization of religious practices found within these urban healthcare contexts pointed to "the resilience of religion within the constructed human habitat," despite the prediction of secularization of societies and the decline of traditional religions (Hegner and Margry 2017, 2). There has also been a proliferation of "new, eclectically created spiritualities, all serving in a partly global subjectification process of religiosity" (2). Cities are vibrant places where religious and non-religious agency has meant formation of new collectives and practices, thus "influencing the very contours of religion and secularization and the interactions between them" (Emerson and Knight Johnson 2018, 15). For example, in London pluralization and choice have been seen in the establishment of the secular congregation, the Sunday Assembly, whose emphasis is on "live better, help often, wonder more" (Bullock 2017), the growth of Black majority churches (Brierley 2013), the instituting of spaces for Muslims to gather across the city to pray, and in the innovation of Christian-centred communities who congregate to do "messy church," employing creativity and the arts to encounter the divine. The location of Vancouver in the Cascadia region, known for its natural beauty, has affected the proliferation of non-religious practices that can involve the natural world. Sociologists Todd Ferguson and Jeffrey Tamburello describe in their study of religion and geography, "Beautiful weather, mountains, and waterfronts are not so much competitors for time with religious affiliations but suppliers for *connections to the sacred*" (their emphasis, 2015, 309). This is also noted by religious studies scholar Paul Bramadat (2018) in his description of "reverential naturalism," which captures how the natural beauty of the Cascadia region can "transfix" and "reconfigure" and inform one's spirituality. Alongside the growth of spiritual practices such as meditation, mindfulness, and yoga, diasporic religious groups have grown in their presence, seen in the geographic location of religion on the Highway to Heaven, a three-kilometre stretch of road where more than twenty religious institutions and schools stand side-by-side. It includes Buddhist, Sikh, Hindu, Jewish, and Muslim traditions and Christian churches that are predominantly evangelical Chinese, all combining a blend of English with different global languages (Todd 2013; Dwyer 2017). This multicultural landscape is evidence of how migration and diasporic communities continue to transform Vancouver, even as its natural landscape shapes its propensity toward ecological spiritualities.

Social and religious changes in cities are mirrored in changes in prayer. Just as cities are not fixed spaces, but continually transforming, so are practices of prayer. Prayer is present in religions, spiritualities, and non-religions and is reconfigured when people travel to different spaces and locations (Tweed 2006). Prayer practices are portable resources for making an unknown place home, which are in turn shaped by the context in which they become embedded (Beckford 1989;

Tweed 2006; Sharma and Guest 2013). Prayer is woven into cities that are "dynamic and heterogeneous socio-cultural, economic and geographic formations" (Hegner and Margry 2017, 7). Prayer all at once can be global and transnational generated by groups and individuals, and shifting as these actors adapt their practices to locality and context. These dynamics contributed to the distinct and plural nature of prayer in our research as people confronted and adjusted to the changing social landscapes of cities that our field sites exemplified and embodied.

Personalization

Prayer in London and Vancouver was not only distinct and plural, but personal, revealing the lived nature of religion in the public sphere. People made prayer their own, personalizing it in their everyday. In the study of religion, since the mid-1980s there has been a "re-centring of 'lived religion'" (Ammerman 2016, 2018). This has opened up explorations of religiosity and non-religiosity where creedal and non-creedal, ancient and modern forms have been examined for their fluidity in everyday life (Baker and Dinham 2017). Nancy Ammerman (2016), in her work on the sociology of religion, explains how lived religion is often defined by what it is not – it is not the study of official spokespersons or formal religious institutions, but rather of the ordinary and mundane, the hidden and supressed who come into view and their stories are told and accounted for. Ammerman states that while this refocusing has been invaluable, a risk of this approach is that it creates a binary by which formal religious communities can be ignored. She proposes widening the study of lived religion to include these groups in order to enrich sociologists' understanding of lived religious beliefs and practices. In our research in London and Vancouver, we observed the ways that prayer was lived and enacted amongst ordinary people in embodied ways, external to official religious institutions. However, chapels, sacred spaces, and prayer rooms where we also observed lived prayer were formally designated domains typically led by official spokespersons (i.e., imams, ordained clergy). Likewise, prayers at the bedside, in addition to informal modes, were often made formally religious and spiritual (e.g., Holy Eucharist or Anointing of the Sick). For the chaplains in our study, prayer was a "comfort zone." For many of the healthcare professionals, while they might pray privately or personally, prayer in healthcare settings was out of place, as the sacred received little acknowledgment in a biomedical world. Thus healthcare settings in London and Vancouver were unique for the study of lived prayer because of how these spaces were a mixture of official and unofficial, biomedical and spiritual, rational and embodied, formal and informal, public and private. Expressions of prayer and those who prayed often occupied a liminal state between these poles, which meant the binary that Ammerman sheds light on was frequently transgressed, operating between the centre and the margins.

Politicization

At our research sites in London and Vancouver, prayer was not without politicization, demonstrating that religion in the public sphere continues to be a vehicle for peace and antagonism. Ammerman (2018) contends that the recentring of lived religion has brought into view the rise of other faiths and non-religions. This is in large part because of migration flows and the decline of majoritarian religions in the running of institutions such as schools, government, and hospitals. Yet the regard for non-majoritarian faiths and non-religions is entangled with relations of power, and processes of inclusion and exclusion that operate along axes of racialization, classism, sexism, and homophobia. With super-diversity in cities like London and Vancouver, difference for many is marked by religion, race, gender, sexuality, ability, age, and class. "Whether it is skin colour or forms of dress, visible signs mark Muslims in Europe and the US as 'other.' Those marks then define both the macro structures of law and citizenship the micro-structures of everyday interaction" (Ammerman 2018, 107).

Vestiges of empire are enacted through these structures, whereby prayer can be dismissed as cultural difference because it is associated with the Other, observed in how Indigenous and migrant communities' traditions have been treated and denied through racialization and sexism, or in the case of Muslim faith communities, Islamophobic stereotypes associated with terrorism and securitization. The result of transatlantic flows of migration, established majoritarian religions have been disrupted by the increase of non-Christian religions and non-white Christians, many of whom are leading Christian churches. It is becoming more common that the racialized body of the Other has transgressed the centre from the margins to be in a position of prominence. Practices of prayer become a complicated mix of culture and power. This raises questions of who gets to pray, who gets space to pray, and who gets time to pray.

Included in these questions about the politicization of prayer are the non-religious. How are their needs for prayer provided for in spaces of healthcare? What exactly are those needs? One of our chaplains asked, "How do we provide for the non-religious?" Sociologists of religion have recently begun to research this rising demographic (e.g., Beaman, Steele, and Pringnitz 2018; Drescher 2016; Lee 2015; Woodhead 2017). Linda Woodhead (2017) reports from her research in the United Kingdom that the non-religious are both "like and unlike religion" and committed to "freedom, diversity and loving-kindness," can hold commitments that are "deeply consumerist to deeply ecological," and are strongly against the sexual abuse by the church (261). As such, researching the nones has pushed sociologists of religion "into the broader realm of culture and values" (262). In the sites we studied, participants felt that they could provide for the non-religious because of the person-centred approach of chaplains and the inclusive values each healthcare setting upheld, espousing a place for everyone and where everyone is respected. This conviction must be located in the context of healthcare where majoritarian religion in Canada and England holds little sway as a monolith, although vestiges of privilege remain, and majoritarian religion enters via individuals. The challenges in these contexts that we studied were the assumptions made about 'no-religion' at point of admission, some users not declaring their non-religious identities because of being in a secular or religious-affiliated hospital, the wide variation of what non-religious means in practice, and what their actual needs for prayer might be. Thus the non-religious, while growing in number, could make up a minority voice among participants and their needs for prayer hidden among hospital users. In London and Vancouver, where there are a range of faith traditions and none, expressions of prayer demonstrated that religion in the public sphere could be all at once contested, highly visible, lack representation, misunderstood, sidelined, acknowledged, and embraced, demonstrating that prayer, and religion, is not only plural and personal but also political.

WHAT DOES THE STUDY OF PRAYER
OPEN US UP TO?

Prayer as transgression offered a window onto religion in the public sphere and opened us up to the unknown. It unsealed the fact that there is much beyond human experience and human control. This was evidenced in participants requesting prayer before and on the way to surgery and surgeons making time for this. Illness often brings life's fallibility to the fore, and prayer could be a comfort when one is faced with the undetermined outcome of medical procedures. Prayer opened our participants up to the transcendent and metaphysical that were not only set apart from the ordinary, but simultaneously woven into everyday temporalities and spaces of work and service.

Prayer opened participants up to the unknown and also to each other. Where prayer has often been thought to be a private act, it is actually de-privatized in the public sphere of healthcare. Feminist philosopher Judith Butler states, "Very often religion functions as a matrix of subject formation, an embedded framework for valuations, and a mode of belonging and embodied social practice" (2011, 72). The richness of religious lives spills over through requests and acts of prayer. These seep in and become part of secular medical contexts that are linked to the state by government policies, funding, and equality legislation (Beckford 2012). Prayer could, however, disrupt the social order of things, such as the organizing structures of clinical guidelines and procedures, as exemplified in groups requesting spaces for prayer, or individuals not going to surgery until a request for prayer had been granted. Addressing these situations demonstrated another kind of equality at work, that of deep equality where navigating difference led to finding common ground, and acts of recognition and kindness with one another (Beaman 2017a). In fostering deep equality, the focus was on relationships and agonistic respect. In this way prayer could open participants to the unknown of living well together, seen in the pile of shoes of Muslims who had gathered to pray in the Christian chapel or in the religiously and spiritually diverse group of staff who gathered to pray and bless the room of a patient who had died. And while clinical settings have structuring routines, procedures, and policies, personal experiences of being confronted with the unknown in these spaces meant that prayer evoked human agency that reached across borders of difference and power. Agential acts of prayer revealed how participants created meaning, connection, and influence in the public space of healthcare that are situated in "complex, pluralistic and secularising societies" (Ganiel 2017, 80). The act of crossing over, transgressing, and disrupting by prayer could "configure new ways of being and knowing and to plot the different metaphysics that are needed to move away from living alterity premised in difference to living intersubjectivity premised in relationality and solidarity" (Alexander 2005, 8).

WHAT DOES THE STUDY OF PRAYER POINT US TOWARD?

What does our study on prayer point us toward? In the twentieth century, the presence and decline of majoritarian religion in the West was the key issue of investigation. Now, in the twenty-first century, contemporary changes in religion and society are frequently understood through the decline of majoritarian religions, increased flows of migration, the ubiquity of religions and spiritualities in the everyday, and the rise of non-religion. The story of prayer in the midst of this religious change could be understood as one of heightened visibility among religious Others and invisibility among the non-religious. Yet, from our participants, we have learned that prayer encompasses a range of expressions that reflect societal transformations and point toward a few areas for future consideration.

First, the multiplicity of prayer practices does not mean prayer has lost its essence of sociality and connection to something beyond oneself. This remains a constant, as we have observed in our study. Prayer carries its essence forward and reinvents itself, based on shifting personal and societal circumstances. It is continuously transcendent, special, and transforming.

Second, despite the adherence to Christianity declining in the West, people still pray (Bullivant 2017). The how and what of people's prayers is being made sense of by historians, theologians, sociologists, anthropologists, chaplains, lawyers, and health studies scholars. The study of prayer points toward new interdisciplinary sites and synergies and helps us to understand social and religious change from different angles.

Third, clinical settings such as hospices, long-term care facilities, and hospitals are institutions of service and science and domains that have not had sustained scrutiny by social theorists. The social sciences and humanities have a lot to offer healthcare administration, such as with insights into how majoritarian religions keep a foothold on power through heritage, education, and leadership, and corporate health-care identities. In turn, healthcare settings are sites of civil society and social change that social scientists and humanities scholars can learn from, especially about religion, non-religion, and prayer. As illustration, one topic for exploration might be how non-religious requests for prayer are shaping how chaplaincy is transforming in how it is now practised and understood.

Fourth, alternative forms of healing have already crept into state-run health systems (Woodhead 2012), seen in the inclusion of therapeutic practices, contemporary arts practices, and nature. The fostering and preservation of the non-human has grown in societal importance and will become more prominent in healthcare. This trend is seen in the architectural design of new hospital buildings in Canada that have incorporated considerations of the environment and the status of nature into their sacred spaces to recognize Indigenous peoples' histories and relationships to the land. Therapeutic landscapes for healing that consider and include green and blue spaces and animal life are those in which prayer may abound even more among the religious and non-religious, challenging and informing the historical biomedical and secular ethos of these public spaces. Likewise, with religious individuals and groups moving through healthcare systems, how clinical sites design and sustain therapeutic religious landscapes of care and belonging are important.

Fifth, our study of prayer exposed the macro-economics of healthcare and how this could affect the resourcing of prayer and spiritual care for patients, families, and staff. Many of our chaplains agreed that their supportive and pastoral work with staff helped to facilitate their good practice of care. Yet when there is a culture of fiscal constraint, it can affect the spiritual well-being of healthcare staff and administrators, affecting their abilities to provide for patients and to care and mentor each other. "Spiritual pain and suffering" amongst healthcare staff needs further examination and understanding (Quinn 2012, 2017). Related to this are the invisible labours of care carried out by cleaners, morticians, receptionists, security guards, and cafeteria staff. On visits to one research site, we sometimes saw the manager of the news agent next door to the hospital wheeling a trolley of confectionary and magazines into the hospital and up to the wards for patients. This gave those bed-bound a connection to the life of the street and to the world going on outside. What might their stories be on the care of patients, families, and staff? How might the privilege we gave to particular voices in our study of prayer and religion in the public sphere be complemented and augmented by those whose work is often obscure and integral to the everyday running of healthcare settings? Our study of prayer moreover assisted us in noting the existential distress in the provision of care and inequalities in the process of research.

Sixth, how does a study on prayer as transgression push theoretical understandings of transgression? In many ways, it picks up the threads of scholars before us (e.g., Durkheim, Mauss, Bataille, Leiris, Callois, Foucault, Taussig) who were interested in the transgressive and social aspects of the sacred and its presence in the everyday (Hejduk 2010). Others have since come along within the social sciences and humanities to investigate the official and unofficially sacred amid the extraordinary and mundane (e.g., Kong 2001, 2010; McGuire 2008; Orsi 2003). Understanding transgression through prayer interrogates binary understandings of transgression. For example, Bataille saw that prohibitions structure transgression (Hejduk 2010) and in healthcare the secular and clinical can structure the transgressive act of prayer. But transgression is not simply the division between good or bad, or simply a negative, as sometimes understood. "Transgression leads to moments of upheaval and disruption that can lead to new possibilities" (Richman 2002, 15, as quoted in Hejduk 2010, 284). Transgression viewed through the lens of prayer in healthcare revealed that the sacred and profane, religious and secular, public and private exposed and blurred into one another, forging new and unexplored terrain. Applying the theoretical vantage point of transgression uncovered that the sacred has not disappeared with secularization but continues to exist, disrupt, and transform because of its ties to the social and its ability to "cross and dwell" (Tweed 2006). When we attempt to enforce boundaries or limits on the sacred, the social plays a part in diminishing them in order that the sacred, or prayer, may occur, therefore upsetting and offering opportunities for well-being and equality in healthcare settings. Examining the mutual shaping of prayer and transgression in healthcare, moreover, unearths agential acts that resist structures of power and manifest forms of release that expose the vulnerability of who we are and what we need.

Finally, asking participants about "prayer as transgression" uncovered pressing issues about religion that have been with us and that will continue to be with us. Prayer as transgression showed us how contentious and provocative religion is in the public sphere. It pointed to the social, institutional, and individual boundaries that limit religion and that religion crosses. It unveiled structures of power and privilege, and the marks of colonialism and patriarchy that intersect and run deep. It exposed participants' loyalties to their faith and its significance to their lives. Multiple expressions of prayer crossed the religious bounds by which they have been historically perceived and contained, revealing mobile and transient, informal and unscripted modes of prayer. Prayer as transgression uncovered the importance participants placed on everyone belonging, and the fear and realities of being marginalized and excluded because of one's religion or non-religion. Asking about prayer as transgression got to the concealed labour of care and deep equality that happens among people of all walks of life. Studying prayer as transgression turned up typical and unlikely spaces where practices of various faiths occur and how bodies, arts, and nature play a role too. The power of prayer pointed us toward how religion and non-religion are being navigated, contested, accepted, and transformed in the public sphere. Prayer transgressed biomedical power, creating more democratic spaces that are evidence of deep equality at work and that accommodate different perspectives on care. Thus prayer was only part of the story of our participants' lives, and yet issues that mattered deeply to them and to today's world were embedded in the social relations of prayer in healthcare.

Research Methods

Brenda Corcoran Smith, Sheryl Reimer-Kirkham,
and Sonya Sharma

This study, *Prayer as Transgression?*, began with a pilot project that explored how social processes shape everyday expressions of prayer in long-term care home sites (Reimer-Kirkham and Sharma et. al. 2018). We launched the pilot study in 2014 to test the feasibility of our data collection methods. With a good measure of reassurance that our methods were suitably designed, we commenced the international, multidisciplinary research project that explored prayer in London and Vancouver healthcare settings in the autumn of 2015. Collectively, these two studies formed what the research team conveniently dubbed The Prayer Project.

From my (Brenda Corcoran Smith) perspective as research coordinator, I was struck with the breadth and magnitude of this qualitative study, the calibre of the research team and its academic collaborators, and the depth and richness of the participants' stories. This was a complex project with many moving pieces. Across twenty-one research sites, located in Vancouver, Canada, and London, England, we conducted 159 interviews (25 from our pilot project); photographed dozens of sacred spaces (formal and informal), artifacts, artworks, and surrounding nature; collected and analyzed twenty-four participant research diaries; and reviewed relevant organizational policies for each of the research sites. We immersed ourselves in our respective research sites over a span of twelve months between May 2016 and May 2017. During this time, the study's co-leads (Sheryl Reimer-Kirkham and Sonya Sharma) spent time in both Vancouver and London research sites. Regular weekly team meetings, bimonthly interna-

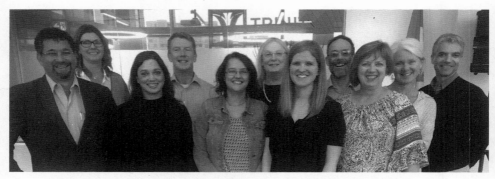

11.1   Research team. *From left to right*: Christopher De Bono, Brenda Corcoran Smith, Sonya Sharma, Barry Quinn, Melania Calestani, Christina Beardsley, Rachel Brown, Andrew Todd, Sheryl Reimer-Kirkham, Lori G. Beaman, Paul Bramadat. Missing: Sylvia Collins-Mayo.

tional team meetings, meeting minutes, and a heap of activity spread-sheets kept us on task and moving forward.

Reimer-Kirkham, based at Trinity Western University in Langley, British Columbia, and Sharma at Kingston University in London, England, led the team of multidisciplinary researchers and academic collaborators from the disciplines of sociology, anthropology, theology/chaplaincy studies, religion, and nursing. The highlight for me was the gathering of this highly regarded scholarly crowd for the project's think tank, a three-day event held in September of 2017 in Richmond, British Columbia. Sonya Sharma, Christina Beardsley, Melania Calestani, Barry Quinn, and Andrew Todd, travelled from London, and Lori G. Beaman, Rachel Brown, Paul Bramadat, Christopher DeBono, Sheryl Reimer-Kirkham, and Brenda Corcoran Smith, arrived from other parts of Canada, while Sylvia Collins-Mayo of London joined us via video-conferencing. Our distinguished collaborators generously provided their scholarly expertise and maximized the project's theoretical and practical contribution (see figure 11.1).

ACCESS AND PARTICIPANTS

Our investigation across international research sites required the time-intensive and detailed completion of six institutional ethics reviews (regional health authorities, universities, a national health system). With all ethics reviews approved, we proceeded with data collection. Our pilot project proved beneficial in accessing the research sites for our *Prayer as Transgression?* study. In Canada, we conducted a pilot project on prayer in long-term care homes. In doing so, we formed important working relationships with key leadership contacts from our healthcare settings. Also, as part of the pilot project, Sharma conducted three interviews with chaplains in London to gain a better sense of how our data collection methodology would work within an international setting (Reimer-Kirkham and Sharma et al. 2018). This proved to be an invaluable experience as it linked us with Christina Beardsley, a lead chaplain who was able to arrange participant access at our healthcare settings in England. Such an auspicious meeting really, as our initial collaborating site fell through earlier that same day!

The twenty-one settings comprised four acute care hospitals (ranging in number of beds from 100 to 430, two in each city); one hospice; two street clinics; and fourteen long-term care centres. We aimed to recruit seventy participants (thirty-five from both cities) for our sample. Because of the number of people keen to contribute to our project, we interviewed ninety-four participants (fifty in Vancouver, forty-four in London). Our purposive sample comprised five participant groups: chaplains (referred to as spiritual health practitioners in the Canadian context and spiritual care professionals in the British context); spiritual care volunteers; administrators at various organizational levels; citizens (former patients or family members of former patients); and healthcare professionals. For a numerical breakdown of each category, please see table 11.1. In addition, another fifteen chaplains and administrators participated in our pilot project (twelve in Vancouver, three in London) for a total of 109 participants across the two studies. As noted in the Introduction, chaplains served as our entrée to the project; together with the spiritual care volunteers, they represent 40% of the sample, balanced with representation from healthcare professionals (23%), administrators (20%), and citizens/family/former patients/residents (17%). This mix of participants has allowed us to construct an interprofessional, multiperspectival portrayal of the social relations of prayer, well beyond what a study of prayer in hospitals as viewed by chaplains alone might offer. We were aiming for more first-hand accounts from patients and former patients, but found this a particularly difficult group to recruit, given the limitations placed on us by research ethics protocol. Also as possible limitation, our research sites may not be as representative of contexts where publicly funded healthcare is not the primary model.

In both London and Vancouver, more females than males participated (with an approximate ratio of three women for every two men).

Table 11.1   Sample demographics

Demographic characteristic	Vancouver (n = 50)	London (n = 44)	Pilot (n = 15)	Total (n = 109)
Roles (n = 109)				
Chaplain	13	8	11	32
Spiritual care volunteer	4	8	–	12
Healthcare professional	18	7	–	25
Administrator	8	10	4	22
Citizen/family/former patient/resident	7	11	–	18
Religious affiliation, self-identified (n = 109)				
Christian	35	22	11	68
Catholic	17	7	–	24
Church of England / Anglican	1	7	–	8
Christian (non-specific)	5	5	4	14
Baptist	1	–	3	4
Evangelical	1	–	–	1
Protestant	1	–	–	1
Presbyterian	2	–	–	2
Pentecostal	2	2	2	6
Mennonite	1	–	–	1
Seventh Day Adventist	1	–	–	1
Quaker	1	–	–	1
Orthodox	1	1	–	2
Salvation Army	–	–	2	2
First Nation Christian	1	–	–	1
Minority religion	6	10	1	17
Jewish	–	1	1	2
Muslim	2	5	–	7
Sikh	1	1	–	2
Buddhist	1	–	–	1
Hindu	1	3	–	4
Baha'í	1	–	–	1
Non-religious	4	10		14
None	4	6	–	10
Spiritual	–	1	–	1
Pagan	–	1	–	1
Atheist	–	1	–	1
Humanist	–	1	–	1
No response	5	2	3	10
Ethnicity, self-identified (n = 94)				
African	–	6		6
African-Caribbean	1	2		3
Asian	8	1		9
Middle Eastern	1	–		1
Southeast Asian	5	5		10
North American (Canadian, USA)	9	–		9
Indigenous	3	–		3
European	17	29		46
Central American	1	–		1
South American	–	1		1

Based on the participants' self-identified reports on ethnicity and faith affiliation, we recruited a relatively diverse sample as displayed in table 11.1. However, the table's depiction does not capture the fluidity and hybridity of identities, such as one participant who identified as South American, African, Caribbean, and Islamic. In these circumstances, we selected the participant's initial response (i.e., South American in the example above), when aggregating ethnicities. Overall, 52% of the sample identified their ethnicity as emanating from Europe, while 26% of the sample self-identified as Asian (China, South Asia, Southeast Asia) or the Middle East. The remaining 22% of participants identified ethnicities as African, Latin, Indigenous, or North American. Ethnic diversity was greater in Vancouver than London (i.e., with a larger number self-identifying as other than North American or European heritage), whereas religious diversity was greater in London (e.g., with larger numbers identifying as other than Christian affiliated).

Of note is the within-group diversity and ecumenical nature of those identifying as Christian (see table 11.1). There was a range of Christian identities represented across the research sites in Vancouver and London: for example, evangelical Christian, Catholic, Anglican, Quaker, Seventh Day Adventist, and Pentecostal. In Vancouver, 12% of the sample identified with a minority religion. In London, 23% of the sample identified with a minority religion. From both sites, some participants identified as no religion or nones. In Vancouver, 8% of participants self-identified as none ($n = 4$), a percentage that is considerably less than the current profile of non-religious affiliation in that city. The number of nones in London was higher, with 23% ($n = 10$) indicating none or some other non-religious identity (e.g., Pagan, Humanist, or Atheist).

We assigned pseudonyms to each of the participants involved in this study to ensure participant confidentiality. In addition to assigning pseudonyms, further de-identifying measures were exercised if there was a concern that the individual participant was at risk of being identified by collateral details contained within the book. Care was taken to ensure that any alterations in identity did not affect the meaning ascribed to the data. Also, as part of our commitment to ethics and participant confidentiality, as a team we chose to make our research sites anonymous. Inevitably, there are benefits and risks to naming research sites. Some general benefits are that it can help to initiate institutional change in relation to organizational policies and highlight examples of good practice particular to institutions that others can learn from. A general and significant risk of naming research sites is that participant confidentiality is potentially revealed, even though each participant will have gone through a process of blinding, as explained above. Our efforts have been to maintain ethical principles and procedures, while offering readers rich and critical analyses of the politics and complexities of the social relations of prayer in healthcare settings.

Using critical ethnography for its ability to uncover how social processes shape the everyday, we captured how prayer was expressed in public institutions (using healthcare as exemplar) through extensive and innovative participatory fieldwork with interviews, observations, photography, and focus groups. Participant recruitment was facilitated through clinical collaborators across our respective Vancouver and London research sites. The clinical collaborators distributed our research project brochure or an email message to potential participants. Interested participants contacted the project coordinator or other members of the research team. Informed consent was acquired from each of the study's participants in advance of data collection, and in the case of the chaplain participants, ongoing consent (also known as process consent) was sought throughout the research project. Three chaplains withdrew from the study following completion of the initial interview. One Vancouver chaplain withdrew, citing time constraints, while one London chaplain withdrew for health reasons and another due to time constraints.

The chaplains participated in a series of three interviews over a twelve-week period, conducted in their workplaces (i.e., hospitals, long-term care homes, clinics). The initial interview served to establish rapport, while gathering data related to the role of the chaplain and the definition, form, and content of prayer. Also, during the initial interview, researchers asked the chaplains to keep a research diary with a minimum of three entries over a period of six weeks, to describe how they enacted prayer and the relationships and contexts in which prayer occurred. This particular method of data collection provided us with a more intimate understanding as to how prayer is framed by and transgresses social and institutional norms. Diary entries provided chaplains the opportunity to engage as "collaborators in the construction of the account" while offering insight and meaning into ordinary, everyday sequences of events (Alaszewski 2006; Elliott 1997; Harvey 2011). We provided each of the chaplain participants with a set of research diary guidelines and prompts to assist them with this process. For example, *Describe the situation in which prayer occurred. What were your thoughts/feelings as you offered prayer? What facilitates the practice of prayer? What makes it more difficult?*

The second interview was a walking interview led by the chaplain participant. These walking interviews strengthened the ethnographic nature of our data collection, as participants had more control over the content of the interview conversation and chose what they wished to show the researchers to best typify their reality (Clark 2010). We asked to show us places important to their work and where prayer occurred. The walking interviews presented opportunity for researchers to make observations of the institutional context (practice environment) permitting deeper elicitation about the everyday, as well as unexpected insights about events or spaces in which prayer occurred. Many of the photographs of prayer spaces, religious icons, symbols, signage, and artwork gathered for data collection were acquired during these walking interviews.

The third and final interview sought to explore how chaplains accommodate and resist institutional healthcare conventions, relations of power, and social differences. Researchers also elicited chaplain recommendations related to practice, policies, and resources for spirituality in healthcare settings. Over the course of three interviews, researchers grew more aware of our shifting positionalities. As expressed in the field notes of one researcher (Sandra), "The ambiance is relaxed – it is like greeting a friend, since rapport was established in interview 1 and 2, I reflect that this is the nice part of a 3rd interview." With multiple encounters, the participant-researcher binary became less distinct and more fluid as a result of the complexity of the participants' and researchers' lived realities and experiences and how they manifested in relationships and interactions with one another (Sharma, Reimer-Kirkham, and Cochrane 2009). Information gathering was not a unilateral activity. Within her field notes, another researcher (Sheryl) revealed, "As with some other interviews, this person [participant] said the interview made him more thoughtful and gave him some ideas about future hospital visitations." Also embodying this collaborative and relational experience, some chaplains took it upon themselves to share with us their personal artistic works that reflected the profound meaning they ascribed to their work (e.g., written poetry, painted artwork, and blog posts).

In addition to the data collection with chaplains, we conducted in-depth, semi-structured interviews lasting for approximately one hour with administrators, healthcare professionals (e.g., nurses, social workers, physiotherapists, doctors), and citizens (e.g., community faith leaders, former patients, and families). These additional interviews were critical in gaining the broad picture of prayer in healthcare settings portrayed in the preceding chapters.

During the initial stages of the study, we established a Practice Advisory Group (PAG) consisting of interested stakeholders for Vancouver and London research sites. In total, six PAG meetings were held, three in Vancouver (April 2016, January 2017, February 2018) and three in London (September 2016, March 2017, March 2018). The purpose of the PAG was to advise on the project to ensure its practical relevance. This included framing some of the research questions to ensure they were relevant to their respective settings; to assist with logistics such as access to the research sites and recommended recruitment strategies; and eventually, to provide us with their ideas for mobilization of research findings. PAG meeting contents were included in our data set as focus groups. Some of the valuable input gathered from our PAG meetings included the recommendation of a shortened project title in Vancouver ("The Expression of Prayer") and a stronger integration of culture, particularly Indigenous culture, in considering religion and spirituality in Vancouver.

DATA ANALYSIS AND REFLEXIVITY

Given the geography of the project and for any organized form of data analysis to occur, a comprehensive data management system was necessary. All data were stored on a secured, password-protected web interface or cloud platform so that the core members of the Canadian and British research teams had access to the accumulated data. Upon completing each of the recorded participant interviews, audio files were transcribed, reviewed for accuracy, and de-identified. We uploaded the de-identified transcripts to NVivo™ 11, a software program for qualitative data analysis. In addition to the interview transcripts, we uploaded project photographs, chaplain research diaries, and observational field notes to NVivo™ 11. Guided by the study's objectives, the theoretical perspectives informing this work, and the interview questions, we generated a detailed codebook (entered as nodes in NVivo™ 11). As the initial codebook and conceptual structure was established, further data collection clarified, verified, and expanded it. The final version of the codebook consisted of nineteen pages with twenty-four parent nodes and 106 subcategories (or sub-nodes). In part, the expansive codebook was the product of an interdisciplinary team effort and the multiple viewpoints it proffered. With so many nodes and subcategories, the need for descriptions and examples for each became evident. For example, the parent node "Prayer – expressions, forms of" held a number of subcategories. Temporal prayer was one such subcategory and was defined as "moments when prayer occurs." Examples of temporal prayer included prayer "near end of life; before meals; before meetings; before surgery or procedure." These descriptors and related examples assisted researchers with coding in a consistent manner, thereby enhancing the reliability of our analysis. A memo entitled "end-of-life care spiritual care" was created as a place in which coders could track analytic observations related to spiritual care at the intersection of death and dying.

Using NVivo™ 11, we were able to compare data across interviews and retrieve exemplars of node categories; in this way, the software facilitated analysis through evolving levels of abstract meaning with thematic analysis. Thematic analysis based on the data-driven inductive approach was undertaken (Braun and Clarke 2006, 2014). The analysis involved an iterative and reflective process. Themes were identified through reading and re-reading transcripts. Transcripts were initially read and coded independently by researchers into themes and sub-themes with regular discussion and revision with the overall team. Disagreements were resolved through discussion and themes, and sub-themes were amended accordingly. We used an iterative process between coding and writing. The core research team held regular web-based meetings to discuss all of the data (interviews, research diaries, observational field notes, researcher memos) in relation to the analytic process, creating a composite description of prayer in hospital settings. The significance of information technology for this project cannot be understated. The availability of web-based meetings and storage platforms allowed the international research team to manage space and time across two continents and nine time zones. At key points, co-leads Reimer-Kirkham and Sharma met for intensive periods of data analysis and manuscript writing.

As researchers, we were aware that our individual social locations, beliefs and values, academic disciplines, even what we chose to read, all shaped the questions we asked, what we observed, what we heard, what we interpreted and finally, what we constructed as knowledge. Our field notes and ongoing conversations helped to surface how our respective viewpoints and experiences influenced the analytic processes. Here, the researcher (Christina) documented in her field notes, her thoughts and perceptions following an interview with a citizen:

He was wearing silver earrings and tattoos on his wrists. They conveyed his Indian ethnicity and he spoke passionately about India and Hinduism and warmly of UK multi-culturalism. I would have preferred the interview to have lasted longer and for him to have said more, especially after initial articulate responses to each question in spite of my providing supplementary questions – which were probably not open-ended enough! I suspect his brevity was related to his mental health and felt that he was happy to contribute to the project but that he also valued his privacy and was keen for the interview to be over.

The inclusion of embodied awareness – an epistemological approach consisting of a "trialectic relationship" between the body, self, and society (Hudak, McKeever, and Wright 2007; Soja 2008) – when acknowledged and further explored in the participant and researcher encounter, generates a deeper sense of meaning and substance in the analytic process (Sharma, Reimer-Kirkham, and Cochrane 2009). Sharma and colleagues (2009, 1648) assert, "Failing to account for the ways that we as researchers experience the field and the processes within data gathering can imply a neutrality and position of power that can be exploitive." In this instance Christina was confronted with the tension of wanting to ask more but was in tune with how much the participant was willing and able to give. This was navigated in part through a bodily awareness of hesitation and feeling the space of encounter between them.

The researchers also exercised reflexivity in the form of open memos in NVivo™ 11. These memos provided research team members with the opportunity to contribute their respective observations, insights, developing ideas, and interpretations as the analytic process ensued. Here, the researcher (Rachel) queried the complexities surrounding mental health disorders and spiritual healthcare:

Where is the line between mental health and spirituality, i.e., when is someone offered spiritual healthcare and when is someone offered psychological healthcare? Is it simply a matter of when and where the patient is admitted? Under what circumstances? Does substance use play a role in whether someone's questions and queries are labelled as spiritual ones versus ones indicative of mental health issues?

In asking these questions, Rachel approached the data from a new, emerging perspective that inevitably shifted the depth of her analysis. For example, in the excerpt above she queried the provision of spiritual care versus psychological care for the patient with a mental health disorder. In chapter 6, we saw how Rachel's deeper analysis of the data supported an alternate angle of vision, one that embodies a more integrated care approach for those afflicted with mental illness. Biomedical treatment modalities were, in fact, not always devoid of spiritual care. She discussed how chaplains prudently navigated these complex circumstances in their endeavour to provide spiritual care as part of the patient's holistic care plan.

Throughout this qualitative study, reflexivity was a vital component of the knowledge construction. As researchers, we were more than mere instruments in the research process. We were the embodied constituents that influenced and shaped our study's findings, based on our respective lived experiences. Sharma and colleagues (2009, 1646) concur: "In being an embodied researcher, value-free, objective, stable, secure, and safe research is very much an illusion, as is the notion that one is just a 'researcher' while in the field." Here, the researcher (Melania) documented her personal thoughts following her initial interview with a chaplain participant:

The interview was not very long, and the answers seemed not to convey any emotional side to what prayer meant to the participant. I had the impression the participant prayed because this was what he was supposed to do, a sort of obligation as part of his faith. I don't know if he didn't feel he could share much with me because he didn't know me very well or because I was not [of the same faith] or because I was a woman.

Our visceral responses, when included as part of reflexive research work, are unique to qualitative inquiry and helps to reveal new discoveries within the data that might otherwise remain untapped (Sharma, Reimer-Kirkham, and Cochrane 2009). Our reflexivity extends to project limitations more generally. Perhaps the most prominent limitation is the lack of representation of larger numbers of nones and religions other than Christian, within our sample. Moreover, because of some religiously affiliated research sites in Vancouver, our findings from these cannot be considered generalizable to other Canadian healthcare organizations.

KNOWLEDGE MOBILIZATION

The strategies we employed for knowledge mobilization varied from traditional forms of academic dissemination to engagement with community stakeholders and decision-makers to utilizing digital technologies to expert consultation. In the very early stages of the project, we developed a project blog with reflections from our walking interviews and visual postings about the spaces in which prayer was enacted. Also, during the initial phase of the research project and throughout, the Practice Advisory Groups, both in Canada and England, were presented with preliminary and updated findings. Through the PAGs, we mobilized knowledge at grassroots and local levels. Project leads presented findings to decision-makers at our research sites and other regional health organizations.

Members of the research team delivered scholarly presentations at conferences, seminars, and events. The project findings have been integrated into undergraduate and graduate courses taught by team members. Recognizing that many of those who pick up this book are healthcare clinicians, practitioners, and administrators, we have developed Recommendations for Healthcare (see appendix II) as a further knowledge mobilization strategy.

At the end of the project, we feel a sense of profound gratitude for the 109 participants who graciously gave of their time and voiced such enthusiasm for the project. For the reader, we trust that the project's varied methods, international settings, diverse sample, rich narratives, and insightful analyses offer an engaging window into religion in the public sphere. Most importantly, we hope that the project and this book contribute to deepened regard and more inclusive spaces for patients and staff in today's healthcare settings.

Recommendations for Healthcare

Sheryl Reimer-Kirkham, Sonya Sharma,
and Brenda Corcoran Smith

As a multidisciplinary group of university researchers (sociology, anthropology, theology, chaplaincy studies, religion, and nursing) and healthcare organizational leaders, we sought to explore the ways that prayer is manifest – whether embraced, tolerated, or resisted – in healthcare settings. We found that prayer, although tolerated and supported within secular and faith-based public healthcare organizations, was complex and even tentative on the ground. It was for the most part delivered sensitively. Based on our analysis of participant interviews and Practice Advisory Group meetings with chaplains, administrators and healthcare professionals, we offer the following recommendations.

EMBRACING DIVERSITY AND CULTURAL SAFETY

Throughout our study, chaplains cited person-centredness as core to their work. Such a stance accounts for diversity, fosters cultural safety, and requires self-awareness of one's own social positioning and limitations in knowledge. The following recommendations aim to enhance this approach:

1 Create educational opportunities for chaplains and health-care professionals for equity, diversity, and inclusion training. Incorporate education on structural vulnerabilities and barriers that impact on spiritual, emotional, and physical wellbeing, so that staff can adequately and sensitively respond to patients and families.

2 Provide education for chaplains and healthcare professionals to enhance religious literacy, focusing on those traditions most common in the surrounding community. This should include foundational knowledge about spirituality in the context of health and healthcare, and the spiritual needs and rituals of nones. Such education should also be incorporated into pre-registration education.

3 For Canadian sites, relationship building with Indigenous communities is vital. More work on integrating the spiritual traditions of Indigenous persons and communities is needed both within healthcare delivery and in partnership with existing spiritual care teams.

4 Consider intersecting factors that may necessitate practices that address individual preferences. Patient vulnerability and gender preferences may transgress assumed cultural or religious norms. For example, a female Muslim patient may prefer a female Christian spiritual care practitioner rather than a male imam.

5 Foster relationships with faith leaders in the community, other stakeholders and networks in an effort to enhance spiritual health services for all. Explore the creation of roles such as religious or cultural brokers who could assess social and religious change, using this information to bridge constituent needs with healthcare services.

6 Aim to provide spiritual care in the preferred language of the patient. This will in many cases require the use of interpretation and translation services.

7 Review and adjust the diverse representation of a chaplaincy team, such that a range of identities are included.

CHAPLAINCY PURPOSE AND LEGITIMACY

Chaplains across research sites highlighted a desire to raise their professional profile and augment their legitimacy as members of the multidisciplinary healthcare team. Spiritual care volunteers and community-based faith leaders desired acknowledgment for providing a valuable service within healthcare settings. The following recommendations can strengthen the contributions of chaplaincy:

1 Spiritual care interventions should be understood as part of holistic and clinical care. This requires ongoing professionalization of the discipline.

2 The model of chaplaincy services, grounded in the social composition of its constituency, may require a combination of generic and multi-faith approaches in order to provide spiritual care to all patients, families, and staff.

3 Encourage inclusion of chaplains in multidisciplinary clinical rounds. Not all patients may want chaplain participation, but everyone should have the opportunity to opt in to chaplaincy services.

4 Facilitate access to patient electronic medical records. Without access, spiritual care assessments, interventions, and subsequent evaluations may be left undocumented, or documented as a separate record, thereby negatively affecting the continuity of care. Spirituality as a clinical issue is then less visible.

5 Provide education and information for staff and the public on the role of chaplaincy within healthcare settings.

6 Support the provision of spiritual care throughout the life span, not only in relation to death and dying. Continuing professional education should be equipping staff to provide spiritual support in all clinical areas, integrated into day-to-day healthcare encounters.

7 Create an ethos where all contributors to spiritual health, including community-based faith leaders and spiritual care volunteers, are valued and welcomed. This can be as simple as allowing for a secure place to store personal items while on site or extending invitations to spiritual health team meetings. Multi-faith networks can do much to support healthcare services in general, and spiritual care specifically.

8 Support further research related to spirituality in healthcare settings, including where chaplains take the lead as principal investigators.

(RE)CONFIGURING SPACE

Chaplains, as well as hospital staff, identified a need to create, expand, or reconfigure indoor and outdoor sacred space within their respective healthcare organizations. The following recommendations address how to make sacred space available and accessible:

1 Dedicated sacred spaces are sanctuaries from high-pressured biomedical clinical areas. Religious services and sacred rituals continue to be meaningful in hospital settings and invite prayer. The

provision of a prayer request book facilitates the expression of
spiritual concerns in meaningful, healing ways.

2 Establish measures and procedures that will accommodate a variety of physical and psychological limitations for those patients
seeking to access sacred spaces. Visible and clear signage is an
important aspect to making sacred spaces accessible.

3 Just as the spirit is fluid, so is sacred space. Create spontaneous
sacred space with the use of visual cues (e.g., butterfly decals or
purple dots to signify a temporary repurposed sacred space). The
integration of the performing arts within public spaces of healthcare, such as dance and song, can create occasions of spiritual
expression for some, while the display of fine arts invites meaningful spaces for reflection for others. For many, indoor/outdoor gardens, water features, and soundscapes can generate serene spaces.

4 Consider the aesthetics of a sacred space with the use of colour,
lighting, material artifacts, ventilation, and building materials.
Create inviting and inclusive spaces. Non-religious rituals and services also require space and can create opportunity for spiritual
reflection, meaningful comfort and solace for patients, families,
and staff. Some organizations choose to provide a multi-faith
space; others provide faith-specific space; others provide both. In
either case, intentionality, consultation, and representation are
important in creating an equitable spatial experience.

ORGANIZATIONAL AND STRUCTURAL SUPPORT

How healthcare organizations respond to diversity is vital. From our
study, it was evident that London and Vancouver healthcare organizations set the tone for spiritual care within their respective institutions.
This organizational response is closely tied to government agendas[1]
and resource allocation that can support or dissuade spiritual care provision. The following recommendations guide organizations in the
support of spiritual care services:

1 While prayer may not easily fit into competing organizational
and clinical priorities, our research findings suggest that organizational mission statements and core values can integrate religion
and spirituality as part of holistic care. Whether secular or faith-
affiliated, to support a diverse constituency, healthcare organizations can make more explicit their support of spiritual health and

spiritual care as a core value. This will give permission to those staff with hesitations about spiritual care to support the spiritual beliefs and practices of patients and families.

2 Explicit organizational support needs to be followed up by resource and space allocation so that staff and the environment supports the spiritual beliefs and practices of patients and families.

3 Create policy (or fully implement existing procedures) for collecting and accessing patient data relevant to their belief system and health. Generate a systematic referral process rather than leaving it solely to patients and family members to request, or for chaplains and volunteers to seek out.

4 Resource professionally-trained spiritual care staff. Accurate and comprehensive spiritual assessments are fundamental to safe and effective spiritual care where needs are recognized and adequately addressed.

5 Healthcare professionals should also be educated to provide point-of-care (or primary) spiritual support such as compassionate presence, referrals to spiritual care, and facilitating the practise of religious rituals (e.g., by ensuring patients can attend a religious service or arranging for the visit of a community faith leader).

6 Acknowledge that spiritual suffering within the context of healthcare is not limited to patients and their families but extends to healthcare staff too, as they witness the suffering of others and bring their own personal suffering as part of who they are. Integrate workplace spiritual health as an organizational priority.

Notes

1 We have de-identified the organizations involved with fictionalized names and have de-identified individual participants with pseudonyms and in some cases other changes. We have grouped various health-care professions (e.g., social workers, nurses, and doctors) together, also to anonymize our participants. Spiritual care volunteers, lay clergy, and community faith leaders are included in the umbrella term of *chaplains*. The category of administrator encompasses executives, middle managers, and line managers of various services. With this level of anonymity, we are striving for rich storytelling in context, without attribution to (and identification of) individual sources. As to our citation practice, we provide the role and site of participants the first time they are cited in each chapter. Likewise for citations from the academic literature – the first time we cite authors in a chapter, we provide their full name and discipline.

2 We have talked long about the nomenclature of chaplaincy, whether to use the Canadian reference of *spiritual care practitioner* or the British Columbia terminology of *spiritual health practitioner*. In England, *chaplain* is understood as an inclusive term. To position our work in relation to the emerging field of chaplaincy studies, we have chosen to use *chaplain* and *chaplaincy* as placeholders for these other terms.

3 Indigenous peoples terminology has evolved in Canada with preferences varying among communities. *Indigenous peoples* is a collective noun for First Nations, Inuit, and Metis. (*First Nations* is a term used to identify Indigenous people who are neither Metis nor Inuit; Metis peo-

ples are of mixed Indigenous and European ancestry; Inuit are Indigenous people in northern Canada.) *Aboriginal peoples* is also a collective
noun to refer to First Nations, Inuit, and Metis peoples and was used in
the Constitution Act 1982. Some First Nations people prefer to not be
called Aboriginal peoples. Many find the term *Indian* derogatory and
outdated, though that term references the legal entity of an Indigenous
person who is registered under the Indian Act. To reflect these preferences, we use the term *Indigenous*, unless directly citing a source with
other terminology. *Indigenous* is capitalized as a sign of respect, the same
way that English and Canadian are capitalized. See Indigenous Corporate Training (2016) for further explanation.

4 Nones are referred to in various ways by scholars and practitioners (e.g.,
nones, Nones, nonreligious, non-religious). For the sake of simplicity, we
have chosen to use *nones* consistently throughout. With this grouping
we cite sociologist Sarah Wilkins-Laflamme, who describes nones as
"individuals who say they have no religion because they either do not
identify with a religious group or tradition, or conventional Western
religious labels do not apply well to them (which is especially the case
for some Indigenous and Asian groups)" (2017a, 2).

CHAPTER ONE

1 In the 2009 case, a community nurse asked an elderly patient during a
home visit if she wanted her to say a prayer for her. The patient com-
plained, and the nurse was suspended without pay for several weeks,
although she was welcomed back to work shortly thereafter (Ahmad
2009). More recently, in November 2016, a nurse was dismissed after
several complaints were made about her "repeatedly talking to patients
about her faith," including offering to pray with patients ahead of
surgery. The dismissal was appealed but subsequently upheld in a May
2019 Court of Appeal ruling (Adams 2019; Rudgard 2017).

CHAPTER TWO

1 There is an extensive literature on the concept of the secular. Some key
contributions to the debates include Berlinerblau (2012), Berlinerblau,
Fainberg, and Nou (2014), Burchardt, Wohlrab-Sahr, and Middell
(2015), Connolly (1999), and Jakobsen and Pellegrini (2008).

CHAPTER THREE

1 There are crosses in each room at some of the religiously affiliated sites (see chapter 8).

2 Smudging is a ceremony practised by some Indigenous peoples of the Americas that involves the burning of sacred herbs, in some cases for spiritual cleansing or blessing.

3 We are aware that there are multiple intersections between class, race, and religion and that these intersections produce different categories of Muslim individuals and communities within the national context in the United Kingdom.

4 See Montemaggi (2015) for a definition of the analytical concept of sacralization. She describes it as the process whereby individual religious actors and groups construct religious tradition by attributing value to single ideas and practices. The concept of sacralization helps us understand how religious actors engage with their religious tradition and participate in constructing it by legitimizing its single elements. The sacred is thus understood as constructed by religious actors as what is of value for them and distinctive of their specific tradition. However, Gilliat-Ray (2010) shows how individuals can engage in personal rituals outside a religious institution to construct informal spirituality through the sacralization of a specific space.

CHAPTER FOUR

1 A consultant report (Bellous 2016) lists anecdotal recommended ratios for chaplaincy care as: hospice/palliative: 1:20 – twenty-five patients; acute: 1:75 patients; long term care: 1:100 patients. Chaplains in British Columbia have informally told us that the average ratio would be much higher in most health organizations. The Working Group BC Spiritual Health Advisory did not provide ratios in their 2012 Report.

2 Canadian healthcare organizations increasingly have Aboriginal Health programs that focus on improving the health of the Indigenous people they serve. These services may include patient navigation, primary care, mental health and substance use services, chronic disease prevention, dental care, and health education.

3 As explained in the Introduction and chapter 2, Canada's national Truth and Reconciliation Commission (2015) addressed Canada's history of

Indian residential schools, with the intent to redress the legacy of residential schools and advance Canadian reconciliation.

CHAPTER FIVE

1 The international call to healthcare chaplains to "develop, implement and document" outcomes (Handzo et al. 2014, 47) relates to their professionalization and adds to an already complex role (see Fitchett 2017, 165).

2 This chapter is one place where our discussion encompasses the United Kingdom, rather than England alone, as in the rest of the book.

3 Named after the late Ken Schwartz, a US healthcare lawyer, who valued the emotional connection during his own dying and left a legacy to found the Schwartz Center, which promotes compassionate care. In the UK Schwartz Rounds are promoted by the Point of Care Foundation to enable all staff, clinical and non-clinical, to explore the emotional and social aspects of working in health care.

4 Note that our use of *specialist* differs in this chapter from how we use it in chapter 6. In this chapter we refer to all chaplains as specialists in spiritual care. In chapter 6 the observation is that chaplains develop specialized knowledge specific to particular clinical areas or population groups (e.g., a chaplain specialized in long-term care).

5 A well-documented dilemma in healthcare chaplaincy history, notably in the three tensions illustrated by Heije Faber's (1971) metaphor of the chaplain as clown, and Paul Prusyer's (1972) belief that by aping other members of the clinical team, chaplains risk betraying their essential vocation (see Beardsley 2006; De Bono 2012, 98–101).

CHAPTER SIX

1 Structural vulnerability is described by anthropologists Bourgois et al. (2017) as the condition of being at risk for negative health outcomes through interface with socioeconomic, political, and cultural/normative hierarchies. People are structurally vulnerable when their location in their society's overlapping and mutually reinforcing power hierarchies (e.g., socioeconomic, racial, cultural) and institutional and policy-level statuses (e.g., immigration status, labour force participation) constrain their ability to access health care and attain health. Healthcare settings themselves can be sites of structural vulnerability, as power hierarchies are in play here too, with accounts of institutional racism and discrimi-

nation against and by healthcare providers (Johnstone and Kanitsaki 2009; Moyce, Lash, and de Leon Siantz 2016; Paradies, Truong, and Priest 2014; Reimer-Kirkham 2003).

2 The concept of personhood has complicated aspects, as reflected in theological, sociological, and philosophic conceptions. For example, see John Swinton's (2012) discussion of personhood in the context of dementia. He argues for a relational understanding of personhood rather than one based on the capacities of a person.

3 See Chris Klassen's (2016) cogent critique of the holism literature in health and disabilities studies, where a "sense of the whole – whether the whole human incorporating mind, body, spirit, or the whole of an ecosystem – tends to place moral implications on anything that represents brokenness or fragmentation.... [I]f, instead of holism, we think of the intra-action of all existence as permeable, still recognizing connectedness in trans-corporeality, we open up the possibilities of present and future flourishing of multiple kinds of materiality" (Klassen 2016, 184).

4 We use the term *long-term care*, as it is the common term in the region of this study. Synonymous terms are *residential care, care homes,* and *nursing homes.* We conducted observations and interviews in eleven different long-term care settings in Canada.

5 *Langar,* a communal meal offered daily at the *gurdwara,* is a central ritual within Sikhism.

6 Beginning in 2013 and skyrocketing in 2016, an unprecedented number of people have died of overdoses in British Columbia as the result of fentanyl, a synthetic opioid, being added to illicit drugs. The high rates of overdose have continued year after year, despite diligent public health measures, and have spread globally. Fentanyl is a less costly but much more potent opioid (10 to 100 times more powerful than heroin). Illicit drug users are generally unaware if a drug is contaminated with fentanyl and die from a lethal dose. See Hayashi et al. 2018; Socías and Wood 2017.

7 While we have included mindfulness meditation as structured prayer here, perhaps our participant would not see it as a prayer practice.

CHAPTER EIGHT

1 *Tayammum,* or dry ablution is the process of performing *wudu* (ceremonial washing or ablution) with sand or soil rather than water. See Rispler-Chaim (2006, 19) and Ze'ev (2005, 142, 167, 232).

APPENDIX TWO

1 In the UK NHS, spiritual care is increasingly included in national health-care policy. In Canada, provinces and regional health authorities vary in the funding provided to spiritual care.

References

Adams, Joel. 2019. "NHS Nurse Who Offered a Bible to a Cancer Patient and Encouraged Him to Sing The Lord Is My Shepherd Loses Appeal after Tribunal Ruled She Was 'Rightly Sacked for Religious Fervour.'" *Daily Mail*, 21 May. https://www.msn.com/en-us/news/uknews/nhs-nurse-who-offered-a-bible-to-a-cancer-patient-and-encouraged-him-to-sing-the-lord-is-my-shepherd-loses-appeal-after-tribunal-ruled-she-was-rightly-sacked-for-religious-fervour/ar-AABGxM7?li=AAaeUIW&%25253Bocid.

Agli, Océane, Nathalie Bailly, and Claude Ferrand. 2015. "Spirituality and Religion in Older Adults with Dementia: A Systematic Review." *International Psychogeriatrics* 27 (5): 715–25.

Ahmad, Ali. 2009. "'Praying Nurse' Returns to Work." *Guardian*, 6 February. https://www.theguardian.com/society/2009/feb/06/petrie-religion-nhs.

Ahmed, Sara. 2012. *On Being Included: Racism and Diversity in Institutional Life*. Durham, NC: Duke University Press.

Alaszewski, Andy. 2006. *Using Diaries for Social Research*. London: Sage.

Alexander, Jacqui M. 2005. *Pedagogies of Crossing: Meditations on Feminism, Sexual Politics, Memory, and the Sacred*. Durham, NC: Duke University Press.

Allen, Chris. 2010. *Islamophobia*. Farnham, UK: Ashgate.

All-Parliamentary Group on Arts, Health and Wellbeing. 2017. *Inquiry Report: Creative Health: The Arts for Health and Wellbeing*. London, UK.

Alzheimer Society of Canada. 2018. "About Alzheimers." http://alzheimer.ca/en/Home/About-dementia.

Ammerman, Nancy T., ed. 2007. *Everyday Religion: Observing Modern Religious Lives*. Oxford: Oxford University Press.

Ammerman, Nancy T. 2016. "Lived Religion as an Emerging Field: An Assessment of Its Contours and Frontiers." *Nordic Journal of Religion and Society* 29 (2): 83–99.

– 2018. "On Things Seen and Unseen: Enlarging the Vision in the Sociology of Religion." In *Foundations and Futures in the Sociology of Religion*, edited by Luke Dogget and Alp Arat, 101–14. London: Routledge.

Angus Reid Institute. 2016. "Prayer: Alive and Well in Canada." http://angus
reid.org/wp-content/uploads/2016/05/2016.05.05-Prayer.pdf.

Appadurai, Arjun. 1994. "Commodities and the Politics of Value." In *Inter-
preting Objects and Collections,* edited by Susan M. Pearce, 76–91. London:
Psychology.

ap Siôn, Tania. 2015. "Prayer Requests in an English Cathedral and a New
Analytic Framework for Intercessory Prayer." In *A Sociology of Prayer*, edit-
ed by Giuseppe Giordan and Linda Woodhead, 169–90. Farnham, UK:
Ashgate.

Armstrong, David. 1983. *Political Anatomy of the Body: Medical Knowledge
in Britain in the Twentieth Century*. Cambridge: Cambridge University
Press.

– 1995. "The Rise of Surveillance Medicine." *Sociology of Health & Illness* 17
(3): 393–404.

Back, Les. (2007) 2013. *The Art of Listening*. Reprint, London: Bloomsbury.

Baker, Chris, and Adam Dinham. 2017. "New Interdisciplinary Spaces of
Religions and Beliefs in Contemporary Thought and Practice: An Analysis." *Religions* 8 (16): 1–12.

Balboni, Michael, and John Peteet, eds. 2017. *Spirituality and Religion within
the Culture of Medicine: From Evidence to Practice*. New York: Oxford University Press.

Balboni, Michael J., Christina M. Puchalski, and John R. Peteet. 2014. "The
Relationship between Medicine, Spirituality and Religion: Three Models
for Integration." *Journal of Religion and Health* 53 (5): 1586–98.

Barnes, Trevor, and James Duncan, eds. 2013. *Writing Worlds: Discourse, Text
and Metaphor in the Representation of Landscape*. London: Routledge.

Bartolini, Nadia, Sara MacKian, and Steve Pile, eds. 2018. *Spaces of Spirituality*. London: Routledge.

Bartolini, Nadia, Chris Robert, Sara MacKian, and Steve Pile. 2017. "The
Place of Spirit: Modernity and the Geographies of Spirituality." *Progress in
Human Geography* 41 (3): 338–54.

Beaman, Lori G., ed. 2012. *Reasonable Accommodation: Managing Religious
Diversity*. Vancouver: UBC Press.

– 2013. "The Will to Religion: Obligatory Religious Citizenship." *Critical
Research on Religion* 1 (2): 141–57.

– 2014. "Deep Equality as an Alternative to Accommodation and Tolerance." *Nordic Journal of Religion and Society* 27 (2): 89–111.

– 2017a. *Deep Equality in an Era of Religious Diversity*. Oxford: Oxford University Press.

– 2017b. "Living Well Together in a (Non) Religious Future: Contributions from the Sociology of Religion." *Sociology of Religion* 78 (1): 9–32.

Beaman, Lori G., Cory Steele, and Keelin Pringnitz. 2018. "The Inclusion of Nonreligion in Religion and Human Rights." *Social Compass* 65 (1): 43–61.

Beckford, James A. 1989. *Religion and Advanced Industrial Society*. London: Unwin Hyman.

– 2012. "SSSR Presidential Address Public Religions and the Postsecular: Critical Reflections." *Journal for the Scientific Study of Religion* 51 (1): 1–19.

– 2014. "Re-thinking Religious Pluralism." In *Religious Pluralism: Framing Religious Diversity in the Contemporary World*, edited by Giuseppe Giordan and Enzo Pace, 15–29. Cham: Springer.

Bellous, Ken. 2016. *Alberta Consortium for Supervised Pastoral Care*. Canadian Association for Spiritual Care. https://spiritualcare.ca/flow/uploads/2016/AC-SPE-Report-Feb-17–16.pdf.

Bender, Courtney. 2003. *Heaven's Kitchen: Living Religion at God's Love We Deliver*. Chicago: University of Chicago Press.

– 2008. "How Does God Answer Back?" *Poetics* 36 (5–6): 476–92.

– 2014. "The Architecture of Multi-Faith Prayer: Hospital Multi-Faith Chapels and Prayer Rooms." Reverberations: New Directions in the Study of Prayer. http://forums.ssrc.org/ndsp/2014/08/04/hospital-multi-faith-chapels-and-prayer-rooms/.

Bentzen, Jeanet Sinding. 2020. "In Crisis, We Pray: Religiosity and the COVID-19 Pandemic." Unpublished paper, University of Copenhagen. 30 March. https://mcusercontent.com/50113b987267c95cf5c9d5b4f/files/07e7548c-b1b3-4043-a3fc-5799aa0cc9ca/Bentzen_religiosity_covid.pdf.

Berlinerblau, Jacques. 2012. *How to Be Secular: A Call to Arms for Religious Freedom*. Boston: Houghton Mifflin Harcourt.

Berlinerblau, Jacques, Sarah Fainberg, and Aurora Nou, eds. 2014. *Secularism on the Edge: Rethinking Church-State Relations in the United States, France, and Israel*. New York: Palgrave Macmillan.

Biberman, Jerry, and Joan Marques. 2014. "Influences of Religion on Spirituality in the Workplace." In *Leading Spiritually: Ten Effective Approaches to Workplace Spirituality*, edited by Joan Marques and Satinder Dhiman, 167–78. New York: Palgrave Macmillan.

Bilge, Sirma. 2010. "Beyond Subordination vs. Resistance: An Intersectional Approach to the Agency of Veiled Muslim Women." *Journal of Intercultural Studies* 31 (1): 9–28.

Bingham, John. 2013. "Britons Still Believe in Prayer – and Young Lead the Way, Poll Suggests." *Telegraph*, 26 March. https://www.telegraph.co.uk/news/religion/9953128/Britons-still-believe-in-prayer-and-young-lead-the-way-poll-suggests.html.

Bishop, Claire. 2005. "The Social Turn: Collaboration and Its Discontents." *Artforum* 44 (6): 178–83.

Bourdieu, Pierre. 1977. *Outline of a Theory of Practice*. Cambridge: Cambridge University Press.

‒ 1984. *Distinction: A Social Critique of the Judgement of Taste*. London: Routledge.

‒ 1991. *Language and Symbolic Power*. Cambridge: Polity.

Bourgois, Philippe, Seth M. Holmes, Kim Sue, and James Quesada. 2017. "Structural Vulnerability: Operationalizing the Concept to Address Health Disparities in Clinical Care." *Academic Medicine* 92 (3): 299–307.

Boyarin, Daniel, and Jonathan Boyarin. 1993. "Diaspora: Generation and the Ground of Jewish Identity." *Critical Inquiry* 19 (4): 693–725.

Brah, Avtar, and Ann Phoenix. 2009. "'Ain't I a Woman?' Revisiting Intersectionality." *Journal of Internal Women's Studies* 5 (3): 75–86.

Bramadat, Paul. 2005. "Religion, Social Capital, and 'The Day That Changed the World.'" *Journal of International Migration and Integration/Revue de L'intégration et de la Migration Internationale* 6 (2): 201–17.

‒ 2018. "Beautiful British Columbia vs Friendly Manitoba: Where You Live May Influence Your Spirituality." CBC Radio, 7 January. http://www.cbc.ca/radio/tapestry/sacred-space-1-architecture-and-region-1.4474834/beautiful-british-columbia-vs-friendly-manitoba-where-you-live-may-influence-your-spirituality-1.4474925.

Bramadat, Paul, Harold Coward, and Kelli I. Stajduhar, eds. 2013. *Spirituality in Hospice Palliative Care*. Albany, NY: SUNY Press.

‒ 2013. "Introduction." In Bramadat, Coward, and Stajduhar, *Spirituality in Hospice Palliative Care*, 1–12.

Bramadat, Paul, and Joe Kaufert. 2013. "Religion, Spirituality, Medical Education and Hospice Palliative Care." In Bramadat, Coward, and Stajduhar, *Spirituality in Hospice Palliative Care*, 67–96.

Braun, Virginia, and Victoria Clarke. 2006. "Using Thematic Analysis in Psychology." *Qualitative Research in Psychology* 3 (2): 77–101.

‒ 2014. "What Can "Thematic Analysis" Offer Health and Wellbeing Researchers?" *International Journal of Qualitative Studies on Health and Well-being* 9. https://psycnet.apa.org/record/2014-54266-001.

Brierley, Peter. 2013. *London's Churches Are Growing! What the London Church*

Census Reveals. London City Mission and Brierley Consultancy, 7 August. https://issuu.com/londoncm/docs/london_church_census_2012_report.

British Broadcasting Corporation (BBC). 2013. "Chaplaincy Services Cut in 40% of English NHS Hospital Trusts." 27 June. https://www.bbc.com/news/uk-england-22990153.

British Medical Journal (BMJ). 1991. "Patient's Charter." 303: 1148. https://doi.org/10.1136/bmj.303.6811.1148.

Broderick, Sheelagh. 2011. "Arts Practices in Unreasonable Doubt: Reflections on Understandings of Arts Practices in Healthcare Contexts." *Arts & Health* 3 (2): 95–109.

Brown, Rachel. 2017. "Bread beyond Borders: Food as Evidence for Thomas Tweed's Theory of Religion." *Bulletin for the Study of Religion* 46 (2): 9–18. https://doi.org/10.1558/bsor.33088.

Buch, Elana D. 2015. "Anthropology of Aging and Care." *Annual Review of Anthropology* 44: 277–93.

Bullivant, Stephen. 2017. *The "No Religion" Population of Britain: Recent Data from the British Social Attitudes Survey (2015) and the European Social Survey (2014).* Catholic Research Forum Reports 3, Benedict XVI Centre for Religion and Society, St Mary's University, Twickenham, London. https://www.stmarys.ac.uk/research/centres/benedict-xvi/docs/2017-may-no-religion-report.pdf.

Bullock, Josh. 2017. "The Sociology of the Sunday Assembly: 'Belonging without Believing' in a Post-Christian Context." PhD diss., Kingston University London.

Burchardt, Marian, Monika Wohlrab-Sahr, and Matthias Middell, eds. 2015. *Multiple Secularities beyond the West: Religion and Modernity in the Global Age.* Boston: de Gruyter.

Butler, Judith. 2011. "Is Judaism Zionism?" In *The Power of Religion in the Public Sphere*, edited by Eduardo Mendieta and Jonathan VanAntwerpen, 70–91. New York: Columbia University Press.

Cadge, Wendy. 2012. *Paging God: Religion in the Halls of Medicine.* Chicago: University of Chicago Press.

Cadge, Wendy, and M. Daglian. 2008. "Blessings, Strength, and Guidance: Prayer Frames in a Hospital Prayer Book." *Poetics* 36 (5–6): 358–73.

Cadge, Wendy, and Emily Sigalow. 2013. "Negotiating Religious Differences: The Strategies of Interfaith Chaplains in Healthcare." *Journal for the Scientific Study of Religion* 52 (1): 146–58.

Canadian Association for Spiritual Care (CASC). n.d. "Our History." https://psycnet.apa.org/record/2014-54266-001.

Carrette, Jeremy R., ed. 1999. *Religion and Culture by Michel Foucault*. Manchester: Manchester University Press.

Casanova, Jose. 1994. *Public Religions in the Modern World*. Chicago: University of Chicago Press.

Cassell, Eric J. 1998. "The Nature of Suffering and the Goals of Medicine." *Loss, Grief & Care* 8 (1–2): 129–42.

Cerulo, Karen A., and Andrea Barra. 2008. "In the Name of ...: Legitimate Interactants in the Dialogue of Prayer." *Poetics* 36 (5–6): 374–88.

Chrysikou, Evangelia. 2014. *Architecture for Psychiatric Environments and Therapeutic Spaces*. Amsterdam: IOS.

Clark, Andrew. 2010. "Using Walking Interviews. Realities Toolkit #13." *ESRC National Centre for Research Methods*, 31 August. http://hummedia .manchester.ac.uk/schools/soss/morgancentre/toolkits/13-toolkit-walking-interviews.pdf.

Coble, Richard. 2015. "Recognition and the Fleeting Glimpse of Intimacy: Tracing the Chaplain's Response to Ungrieved Death." *Journal of Pastoral Care & Counseling* 69 (1): 4–12.

– 2018. *The Chaplain's Presence and Medical Power: Rethinking Loss in the Hospital*. Lanham, MD: Lexington Books.

Coleman, Simon, and John Elsner. 1998. "Performing Pilgrimage: Walsingham and the Ritual Construction of Irony." In *Ritual, Performance, Media*, edited by Felicia Hughes-Freeland, 46–65. London: Routledge.

Collins, Patricia Hill. 1990. *Black Feminist Thought: Knowledge, Consciousness, and the Politics of Empowerment*. New York: Routledge.

Collins, Peter. 2015. "An Analysis of Hospital Chapel Prayer Requests." In *A Sociology of Prayer*, edited by Giuseppe Giordan and Linda Woodhead, 191–211. Farnham, UK: Ashgate.

Collins, Peter, Simon Coleman, Jane Macnaughton, and Tessa Pollard. 2007. *NHS Hospital "Chaplaincies" in a Multi-Faith Society: The Spatial Dimension of Religion and Spirituality in Hospital*. Project Report. NHS, Durham, UK: Durham University.

Colorado, Carlos. 2017. "Reconciliation and the Secular." Paper presented at the annual Congress of the Canadian Society for the Study of Religion, Toronto, ON, 27–30 May.

Connell, Sharon, and Christina Beardsley. 2014. "'Hospitality of the Heart – Hospitality for the Human Spirit': How Healthcare Chaplains Can Discover, Create and Offer Spaces for Spiritual Care in the Hospital Setting." *Health and Social Care Chaplaincy* 2 (1): 65–78.

Connolly, William E. 1999. *Why I Am Not a Secularist*. Minneapolis: University of Minnesota Press.

– 2005. *Pluralism*. Durham, NC: Duke University Press.

Corwin, Anna I. 2012. "Changing God, Changing Bodies: The Impact of New Prayer Practices on Elderly Catholic Nuns' Embodied Experience." *Ethos* 40 (4): 390–410.

Crenshaw, Kimberlé. 1989. "Demarginalizing the Intersection of Race and Sex: A Black Feminist Critique of Antidiscrimination Doctrine, Feminist Theory and Antiracist Politics." *University of Chicago Legal Forum* 139, 139–67.

– 2016. "On Intersectionality." Women of the World Festival, 14 March. https://www.southbankcentre.co.uk/blog/kimberl%C3%A9-crenshaw-wow-2016-keynote.

Crompton, Andrew, and Chris Hewson. 2016. "Designing Equality: Multi-Faith Space as Social Intervention." In *Religion, Equalities, and Inequalities*, edited by Dawn Llewellyn and Sonya Sharma, 77–88. London: Routledge.

Csordas, Thomas J., ed. 1994. *Embodiment and Experience: The Existential Ground of Culture and Self*. Cambridge: Cambridge University Press.

Curtice, John, Elizabeth Clery, Jane Perry, Miranda Phillips, and Nilufer Rahim, eds. 2019. *British Social Attitudes: The 36th Report*. London: National Centre for Social Research.

Das, Veena. 2015. *Affliction: Health, Disease, Poverty*. New York: Fordham University Press.

Davidson, Joyce, Liz Bondi, and Mick Smith, eds. 2005. *Emotional Geographies*. Farnham, UK: Ashgate.

Davie, Grace. 2013. *The Sociology of Religion: A Critical Agenda*. London: Sage.

– 2015. *Religion in Modern Britain: A Persistent Paradox*. Oxford: Wiley-Blackwell.

Davis, Kathy, and Dubravka Zarkov. 2017. "EJWS Retrospective on Intersectionality." *European Journal of Women's Studies* 24 (4): 313–20.

Day, Abby. 2011. *Believing in Belonging: Belief and Social Identity in the Modern World*. Oxford: Oxford University Press.

De Bono, Christopher E. 2012. "An Exploration and Adaptation of Anton T. Boisen's Notion of the Psychiatric Chaplain in Responding to Current Issues in Clinical Chaplaincy." PhD diss., University of St. Michael's College at the University of Toronto.

Demerath, Nicolas J., III. 2000. "The Varieties of Sacred Experience: Finding the Sacred in a Secular Grove." *Journal for the Scientific Study of Religion* 39 (1): 1–11.

– 2007. "Secularization and Sacralization Deconstructed and Reconstructed." In *The SAGE Handbook of the Sociology of Religion*, edited by James A. Beckford and Nicholas J. Demerath III, 57–80. London: Sage.

Department of Health (DOH). 2003. *Spiritual and Religious Care: Meeting the Needs of Patients and Staff. Guidance for Managers and Those Involved in the Provision of Chaplaincy-Spiritual Care.* London: Department of Health.

deVelder, John. 1994. "Reviewed Work: Head and Heart: The Story of the Clinical Pastoral Education Movement." Review of *Head and Heart: The Story of the Clinical Pastoral Education Movement* by Charles E. Hall. *Journal of Religion and Health* 33 (3): 281–4.

Dhamoon, Rita, and Olena Hankivsky. 2011. "Why the Theory and Practice of Intersectionality Matter to Health Research and Policy." In *Health Inequities in Canada: Intersectional Frameworks and Practices*, edited by Olena Hankivsky, 16–52. Vancouver: UBC Press.

Dinham, Adam, and Francis Matthew. 2015. *Religious Literacy in Policy and Practice.* Bristol: Policy Press at the University of Bristol.

Donnelly, Laura. 2017. "NHS Should 'Do' God the New Guideline Suggests, with Doctors Urged to Ask the Dying about Their Religious Views." *Telegraph*, 2 March. https://www.telegraph.co.uk/news/2017/03/02/nhs-should-do-god-new-guidance-suggests-doctors-urged-ask-dying/.

Douglas, Mary. 1966. *Purity and Danger: On Concepts of Pollution and Taboo.* New York: Praeger.

Drescher, Elizabeth. 2016. *Choosing Our Religion: The Spiritual Lives of America's Nones.* New York: Oxford University Press.

Duncan, James. 2004. *The City as Text: The Politics of Landscape Interpretation in the Kandyan Kingdom.* Cambridge: Cambridge University Press.

Duncan, James, and Nancy Duncan. 1988. "(Re)reading the Landscape." *Environment and Planning D: Society and Space* 6 (2): 117–26.

Durkheim, Emile. (1915) 2008. *The Elementary Forms of Religious Life.* Translated by Joseph Ward Swain. New York: Dover.

Dwyer, Claire. 2017. "Spiritualizing the Suburbs: New Religious Architecture in Suburban London and Vancouver." In *Spiritualizing the City: Agency and Resilience of the Urban and Urbanesque Habitat*, edited by Victoria Hegner and Peter Jan Margry, 115–29. London: Routledge.

Eccles, Janet Betty. 2014. "The Chaplaincy Experience: Negotiating (Multi-Faith) Time and Space in a Northern English General Hospital." *Journal of Pastoral Care & Counselling* 68 (3): 1–12.

El-Tayeb, Fatima. 2012. "'Gays Who Cannot Properly Be Gay': Queer Muslims in the Neoliberal European City." *European Journal of Women's Studies* 19 (1): 79–95.

Eliade, Mircea. (1959) 1987. *The Sacred and the Profane.* Translated by Willard R. Trask. New York: Harcourt Brace Jovanovich.

Elliott, Heather. 1997. "The Use of Diaries in Sociological Research on Health Experience." *Sociological Research Online* 2 (2): 1–11.

Ellison, Christopher G., and Jinwoo Lee. 2010. "Spiritual Struggles and Psychological Distress: Is There a Dark Side of Religion?" *Social Indicators Research* 98 (3): 501–17.

Emerson, Michael O., and Lenore M. Knight Johnson. 2018. "Soul of the City: The Depth of How the 'Urban' Matters in the Sociology of Religion." *Sociology of Religion: A Quarterly Review* 79 (1): 1–19.

Equality and Human Rights Commission. 2017. "An Introduction to the Equality Act 2010." https://www.equalityhumanrights.com/en/equality-act-2010/what-equality-act.

Espírito Santo, Diana, and Nico Tassi, eds. 2013. *Making Spirits: Materiality and Transcendence in Contemporary Religions.* New York: IB Tauris.

Faber, Heije. 1971. *Pastoral Care in the Modern Hospital.* London: SCM.

Ferguson, Todd W., and Jeffrey A. Tamburello. 2015. "The Natural Environment as a Spiritual Resource: A Theory of Regional Variation in Religious Adherence." *Sociology of Religion* 76 (3): 295–314.

Field, Clive D. 2017. "Britain on Its Knees: Prayer and the Public since the Second World War." *Social Compass* 64 (1): 92–112.

Finlay, Jessica, Thea Franke, Heather McKay, and Joanie Sims-Gould. 2015. "Therapeutic Landscapes and Wellbeing in Later Life: Impacts of Blue and Green Spaces for Older Adults." *Health & Place* 34 (July): 97–106.

Fitchett, George. 2017. "Recent Progress in Chaplaincy-Related Research." *Journal of Pastoral Care & Counseling* 71 (3): 163–75.

Fitchett, George, and Steve Nolan. 2015. *Spiritual Care in Practice: Case Studies in Healthcare Chaplaincy.* London: Jessica Kingsley.

Fleischer, Stefanie, and Mary Grehan. 2016. "The Arts and Health: Moving Beyond Traditional Medicine." *Journal of Applied Arts & Health* 7 (1): 93–105.

Folland, Mark. 2006. *A Review of Some Theoretical Models of Healthcare Chaplaincy Service and Practice.* South Yorkshire NHS Strategic Health Authority, Sheffield.

Ford, David F. 1999. *Self and Salvation: Being Transformed.* Cambridge: Cambridge University Press.

Foucault, Michel. (1973) 2003. *The Birth of the Clinic: An Archaeology of Medical Perception*, 3rd ed. London: Routledge.

Game, Ann. 1997. "Sociology's Emotions." *Canadian Review of Sociology & Anthropology* 34 (4): 385–99.

Ganiel, Gladys. 2017. "Secularisation and De-Institutionalised Religion." In *Foundations and Futures in the Sociology of Religion*, edited by Luke Dogget and Alp Arat, 68–82. London: Routledge.

Garces-Foley, Kathleen. 2013. "Hospice and the Politics of Spirituality." In *Spirituality in Hospice Palliative Care*, edited by Paul Bramadat, Harold Coward, and Kelli Stajduhar, 13–40. Albany: SUNY.

Geertz, Armin W. 2016. "Comparing Prayer: On Science, Universals, and the Human Condition. In *Essays in Honor of Jonathan Z. Smith*, edited by Willi T. Braun and Russell McCutcheon, 113–39. London: Routledge.

Gesler, Wilbert. 1992. "Therapeutic Landscapes: Medical Issues in Light of the New Cultural Geography." *Social Science & Medicine* 34 (7): 735–46.

Gilliat-Ray, Sophie. 1999. "Sector Ministry in a Sociological Perspective." In *Chaplaincy: The Church's Sector Ministries*, edited by Giles Legood, 25–37. London: Cassell.

– 2005. "'Sacralising' Sacred Space in Public Institutions: A Case Study of the Prayer Space at the Millennium Dome." *Journal of Contemporary Religion* 20 (3): 357–72.

– 2010. "Body-Works and Fieldwork: Research with British Muslim Chaplains." *Culture and Religion* 11 (4): 413–32.

Gilliat-Ray, Sophie, Mansur Ali, and Stephen Pattison. 2013. *Understanding Muslim Chaplaincy*. Farnham, UK: Ashgate.

Gilliat-Ray, Sophie, and Mohammed Arshad. 2015. "Multifaith Working." In *A Handbook of Chaplaincy Studies*, edited by Christopher Swift, Mark Cobb, and Andrew Todd, 109–22. Farnham, UK: Ashgate.

Giordan, Giuseppe. 2015. "Introduction: You Never Know. Prayer as Enchantment." In *A Sociology of Prayer*, edited by Giuseppe Giordan and Linda Woodhead, 1–8. Farnham, UK: Ashgate.

Giordan, Giuseppe, and Linda Woodhead, eds. 2013. *Prayer in Religion and Spirituality*. Vol. 4 of *Annual Review of the Sociology of Religion*. Leiden, Netherlands: Brill.

– eds. 2015. *A Sociology of Prayer*. Farnham, UK: Ashgate.

Goffman, Erving. 1963. *Stigma: Notes on the Management of Spoiled Identity*. New York: Simon & Schuster.

Graham, Elaine L. 2002. *Transforming Practice: Pastoral Theology in an Age of Uncertainty*. Eugene, OR: Wipf and Stock.

Greenleaf, Robert K. 2002. *Servant Leadership: A Journey into the Nature of Legitimate Power and Greatness*. New York. Paulist.

Griffith, Derek. M. 2012. "An Intersectional Approach to Men's Health." *Journal of Men's Health* 9 (2): 106–12.

Gunaratnam, Yasmin. 2013. *Death and the Migrant: Bodies, Borders and Care*. London: Bloomsbury.

– 2014. "Morbid Mixtures: Hybridity, Pain and Transnational Dying." *Subjectivity* 7 (1): 74–91.

Habermas, Jürgen. (1962) 1989. *The Structural Transformation of the Public Sphere: An Inquiry into a Category of Bourgeois Society*. Cambridge: MIT Press.

Hall, David, ed. 1997. *Lived Religion in America: Toward a History of Practice*. Princeton: Princeton University Press.

Hall, Eric, Brian Hughes, and George Handzo. 2016. *Spiritual Care: What It Means, Why It Matters in Health Care*. New York: HealthCare Chaplaincy Network. http://files.constantcontact.com/511297de301/1c955cdb-bf40-4bef-bb56-6bce02f51dc5.pdf?ver=1476887863000.

Handzo, George F., Mark Cobb, Cheryl Holmes, Ewan Kelly, and Shane Sinclair. 2014. "Outcomes for Professional Health Care Chaplaincy: An International Call to Action." *Journal of Health Care Chaplaincy* 20 (2): 43–53.

Hartig, Terry, Richard Mitchell, Sjerp De Vries, and Howard Frumkin. 2014. "Nature and Health." *Annual Review of Public Health* 35 (1): 207–28.

Harvey, Laura. 2011. "Intimate Reflections: Private Diaries in Qualitative Research." *Qualitative Research* 11 (6): 664–82.

Hayashi, Kanna, M-J. Milloy, Mark Lysyshyn, Kora DeBeck, Ekaterina Nosova, Evan Wood, and Thomas Kerr. 2018. "Substance Use Patterns Associated with Recent Exposure to Fentanyl among People Who Inject Drugs in Vancouver, Canada: A Cross-Sectional Urine Toxicology Screening Study." *Drug & Alcohol Dependence* 183:1–6.

Hegner, Victoria, and Peter Jan Margry. 2017. "Introduction: Spiritualizing the Urban and the Urbanesque." In *Spiritualizing the City: Agency and Resilience of the Urban and Urbanesque Habitat*, edited by Victoria Hegner and Peter Jan Margry, 2–24. London: Routledge.

Hejduk, Renata. 2010. "Step into Liquid: Rites, Transcendence and Transgression in the Modern Construction of the Social Sacred." *Culture and Religion: An Interdisciplinary Journal* 11 (3): 277–93.

Henderson, Martha. 1993. "What Is Spiritual Geography?" *Geographical Review* 83 (4): 469–72.

Henery, Neil. 2003. "Critical Commentary: The Reality of Visions: Contemporary Theories of Spirituality in Social Work." *British Journal of Social Work* 33 (8): 1105–13.

Hochschild, Arlie R. 2003. *The Managed Heart: Commercialization of Human Feeling*. 20th ed. Berkeley: University of California Press.

Holloway, Julian. 2003. "Make-Believe: Spiritual Practice, Embodiment, and Sacred Space." *Environment and Planning A* 35 (11): 1961–74.

Holloway, Julian, and Oliver Valins. 2002. "Placing Religion and Spirituality in Geography." *Social and Cultural Geography* 3 (1): 5–9.

Holst, Lawrence. 1973. "The Chaplain Today." In *Toward a Creative Chaplaincy*, edited by Lawrence Holst and Harold Kurtz, 3–14. Springfield, IL: Charles C. Thomas.

hooks, bell. 1984. *Feminist Theory: From Margin to Center*. Boston: Beacon.

– 1994. *Teaching to Transgress: Education as the Practice of Freedom*. New York: Routledge.

Hopkins, Peter. 2007. "Young People, Masculinities, Religion and Race: New Social Geographies." *Progress in Human Geography* 31 (2): 163–77.

Hopkins, Peter, Lily Kong, and Elizabeth Olson, eds. 2012. *Religion and Place: Landscape, Politics and Piety*. London: Springer.

Hoskins, Ryan. 2017. "Holy Healthcare: Our Religious Hospitals Problem." *Alberta Views*, 1 April. https://albertaviews.ca/holy-healthcare/.

Howes, David. 2015. "Sensation and Transmission." In *Ritual, Performance and the Senses*, edited by Jon P. Mitchell and Michael Bull, 153–66. London: Bloomsbury.

Hudak, Pamela L., Patricia McKeever, and James G. Wright. 2007. "Unstable Embodiments: A Phenomenological Interpretation of Patient Satisfaction with Treatment Outcome." *Journal of Medical Humanities* 28 (1): 31–44.

Hudson, Rosalie. 2012. "Personhood." In *Oxford Textbook of Spirituality in Healthcare*, edited by Mark Cobb, Christina Puchalski, and Bruce Rumbold, 105–12. Oxford: Oxford University Press.

Humanists UK. n.d. "Pastoral Support for the Non-Religious." http://humanistcare.org.uk/.

Humble, John G., and Peter Hansell. 1974. *Westminster Hospital 1716–1974*. London: Pitman Medical Publishing.

Hüwelmeier, Gertrud. 2017. "Praying in Berlin's 'Asiatown': Religious Place-Making in a Multi-Ethnic Bazaar." In *Spiritualizing the City: Agency and Resilience of the Urban and Urbanesque Habitat*, edited by Victoria Hegner and Peter Jan Margry, 65–80. London: Routledge.

Indigenous Corporate Training. 2016. "Indigenous Peoples Terminology Guidelines for Usage." 20 July. https://www.ictinc.ca/blog/indigenous-peoples-terminology-guidelines-for-usage.

Jakobsen, Janet R., and Ann Pellegrini, eds. 2008. *Secularisms*. Durham, NC: Duke University Press.

Jernigan, Homer L. 2002. "Clinical Pastoral Education: Reflections on the Past and Rupture of a Movement." *Journal of Pastoral Care & Counseling* 56 (4): 377–92.

Jhutti-Johal, Jagbir. 2013. "Understanding and Coping with Diversity in Healthcare." *Health Care Analysis* 21 (3): 259–70.

Johnstone, Megan-Jane, and Olga Kanitsaki. 2009. "The Spectrum of 'New

Racism' and Discrimination in Hospital Contexts: A Reappraisal." *Collegian* 16 (2): 63–9.

Joshi, Khyati Y. 2006. "The Racialization of Hinduism, Islam, and Sikhism in the United States." *Equity & Excellence in Education* 39:211–26.

Kaplan, Rachel, and Stephen Kaplan. 1989. *The Experience of Nature: A Psychological Perspective*. Cambridge: Cambridge University Press Archive.

Karakas, Fahri, and Emine Sarigollu. 2019. "Spirals of Spirituality: A Qualitative Study Exploring Dynamic Patterns of Spirituality in Turkish Organizations." *Journal of Business Ethics* 156:799–821.

Kianpour, Masoud. 2013. "Mental Health and Hospital Chaplaincy: Strategies of Self-Protection (Case Study: Toronto, Canada)." *Iranian Journal of Psychiatry and Behavioral Sciences* 7 (1): 69–77.

King, Stephen D.W. 2007. *Trust the Process: A History of Clinical Pastoral Education as Theological Education*. Lanham, MD: University Press of America.

Kirk, Pamela. 1990. "Time and Prayer." *Liturgy* 8 (4): 8–15.

Kirkpatrick, Bill. 1988. *Aids: Sharing the Pain. Pastoral Guidelines*. London: Darton, Longman & Todd.

Klassen, Chris. 2016. "Complicating the Whole from the Position of a Broken Body: Interactions between Religion, Disability and Material Feminism." In *Religion, Equalities, and Inequalities*, edited by Dawn Llewellyn and Sonya Sharma, 177–85. London: Routledge.

Kleinman, Arthur. 1988. *Illness Narratives: Suffering, Healing, and the Human Condition*. New York: Basic Books.

Kleinman, Arthur, Veena Das, and Margaret Lock. 1997. *Social Suffering*. Berkeley: University of California Press.

Kong, Lily. 2001. "Mapping 'New' Geographies of Religion: Politics and Poetics in Modernity." *Progress in Human Geography* 25 (2): 211–33.

– 2002. "In Search of Permanent Homes: Singapore's House Churches and the Politics of Space." *Urban Studies* 39 (9): 1573–86.

– 2010. "Global Shifts, Theoretical Shifts: Changing Geographies of Religion." *Progress in Human Geography* 34 (6): 755–76.

Lambert, Patricia Dewey, ed. 2015. *Managing Arts Programs in Healthcare*. London: Routledge.

Lee, Jo, and Tim Ingold. 2006. "Fieldwork on Foot: Perceiving, Routing, Socializing." In *Locating the Field: Space, Place and Context in Anthropology*, edited by Simon Coleman and Peter Collins, 67–85. Oxford: Berg.

Lee, Lois. 2015. *Recognizing the Nonreligious: Reimaging the Secular*. New York: Oxford University Press.

Lee, Simon J. 2002. "In a Secular Spirit: Strategies of Clinical Pastoral Education." *Health Care Analysis* 10 (4): 339–56.

Liefbroer, Anke I., Erik Olsman, R. Ruard Ganzevoort, and Faridi S. van Etten-Jamaludin. 2017. "Interfaith Spiritual Care: A Systematic Review." *Journal of Religion and Health* 56 (5): 1776–93.

Lock, Margaret. 1993. "Cultivating the Body: Anthropology and Epistemologies of Bodily Practice and Knowledge." *Annual Review of Anthropology* 22: 133–55.

Luhrmann, Tanya Marie. 2013. "Making God Real and Making God Good: Some Mechanisms through Which Prayer May Contribute to Healing." *Transcultural Psychiatry* 50 (5): 707–25.

Lupton, Deborah. 1998. *The Emotional Self*. London: Sage.

Maller, Cecily, Mardie Townsend, Anita Pryor, Peter Brown, and Lawrence St. Leger. 2006. "Healthy Nature Healthy People: 'Contact with Nature' as an Upstream Health Promotion Intervention for Populations." *Health Promotion International* 21 (1): 45–54.

Marlatt, G. Alan, and Katie Witkiewitz. 2010. "Update on Harm-Reduction Policy and Intervention Research." *Annual Review of Clinical Psychology* 6: 591–606.

Martin, Angela, and Sandra Kryst. 2005. "Ritualization and Place Contagion in Postmodernity." In *Places through the Body*, edited by Heidi Nast and Steve Pile, 207–29. London: Routledge.

Mason, Michael C. 2013. "Making the Sacred Real." In *Prayer in Religion and Spirituality*. Vol. 4 of *Annual Review of the Sociology of Religion 2013*, edited by Giuseppe Giordan and Linda Woodhead, 9–26. Leiden: Brill.

– 2015. "For Youth, Prayer Is Relationship." In *A Sociology of Prayer*, edited by Giuseppe Giordan and Linda Woodhead, 25–48. Farnham, UK: Ashgate.

Massey, Doreen. 1994. *Space, Place and Gender*. London: Polity.

– 2005. *For Space*. Thousand Oaks, CA: Sage.

Masuzawa, Tomoko. 2005. *The Invention of World Religions: Or, How European Universalism Was Preserved in the Language of Pluralism*. Chicago: University of Chicago Press.

Mauss, Marcel. 2003. *On Prayer*. Edited by William S.F. Pickering. Oxford: Berghahn.

McCullough, James. 2015. *Sense and Spirituality: The Arts and Spiritual Formation*. Eugene, OR: Cascade Books.

McCutcheon, Russell. T. 1997. *Manufacturing Religion: The Discourse on Sui Generis Religion and the Politics of Nostalgia*. New York: Oxford University Press.

McFadyen, Alistair. 1990. *The Call to Personhood: A Christian Theory of the Individual in Social Relationships*. Cambridge: Cambridge University Press.

McGuire, Meredith. 2008. *Lived Religion: Faith and Practice in Everyday Life*. Oxford: Oxford University Press.

McSherry, Wilfred. 2001. "Spiritual Crisis? Call a Nurse." In *Spirituality in Health Care Contexts*, edited by Helen Orchard, 107–17. London: Jessica Kingsley Publishers.

Meecham, Pam, and Julie Sheldon. 2013. *Modern Art: A Critical Introduction*. London: Routledge.

"Merger of the Network for Pastoral, Spiritual and Religious Care in Health (NPSRC) and the Chaplaincy Leadership Forum (CLF)." 2017. 24 November. https://static1.squarespace.com/static/58359f279de4bbe7aba10e31/t /5a1d52e0ec212d9bd36073cd/1511871202158/Merger+Press+Release.pdf.

Meyer, Birgit. 2006. *Religious Sensations: Why Media, Aesthetics and Power Matter in the Study of Contemporary Religion*. Amsterdam: Vrije Universiteit.

– ed. 2009. *Aesthetic Formations: Media, Religion and the Senses*. New York: Palgrave Macmillan.

Meyer, Birgit, David Morgan, Crispin Paine, and S. Brent Plate. 2010. "The Origin and Mission of Material Religion." *Religion* 40 (3): 207–11.

Miller, Jean Baker, and Irene Stiver. 1997. *The Healing Connection: How Women Form Relationships in Therapy and in Life*. Boston: Beacon.

Ministry of Health. 2012. *Spiritual Health: A Framework for British Columbia's Spiritual Health Professionals*. Victoria, BC: Government of British Columbia. 25 July. http://www.health.gov.bc.ca/library/publications/year/2012 /spiritual-health-framework.pdf.

Mirza, Heidi Safia. 2013. "'A Second Skin': Embodied Intersectionality, Transnationalism and Narratives of Identity and Belonging among Muslim Women in Britain." *Women's Studies International Forum* 36 (January–February): 5–15.

Mitchell, David. 2015. "Critical Response to Palliative Care Studies: A Chaplain's Perspective." In *Spiritual Care in Practice: Case Studies in Healthcare Chaplaincy*, edited by George Fitchett and Steve Nolan, 263–71. London: Jessica Kingsley.

Mitchell, Richard. 2013. "Is Physical Activity in Natural Environments Better for Mental Health Than Physical Activity in Other Environments?" *Social Science & Medicine* 91 (August): 130–4.

Montemaggi, Francesca Eva Sara. 2015. "Sacralisation: The Role of Individual Actors in Legitimising Religion." *Culture and Religion* 16 (3): 291–307.

Morgan, David. 2012. *The Embodied Eye: Religious Visual Culture and the Social Life of Feeling*. Berkeley: University of California Press.

Mowat, Harriet. 2008. *The Potential for Efficacy of Healthcare Chaplaincy and*

Spiritual Care Provision in the NHS (UK). Aberdeen: NHS Yorkshire and the Humber and Mowat Research.

Moyce, Sally, Rebecca Lash, and Mary Lou de Leon Siantz. 2016. "Migration Experiences of Foreign Educated Nurses: A Systematic Review of the Literature." *Journal of Transcultural Nursing* 27 (2): 181–8.

National Health Service (NHS). 2007. *Standards for NHS Scotland Chaplaincy Services*. NHS Education for Scotland, 4 March. https://www.nes.scot.nhs.uk/media/290156/chaplaincy__standards_final_version.pdf.

– 2015. *NHS Chaplaincy Guidelines 2015: Promoting Excellence in Pastoral, Spiritual & Religious Care*. NHS England, 6 March. https://www.england.nhs.uk/wp-content/uploads/2015/03/nhs-chaplaincy-guidelines-2015.pdf.

National Health Service National Institute for Clinical Excellence (NICE). 2004. *Guidance on Cancer Services. Improving Supportive and Palliative Care for Adults with Cancer: The Manual*. London: NICE.

Naylor, Simon, and James R. Ryan. 2002. "The Mosque in the Suburbs: Negotiating Religion and Ethnicity in South London." *Social & Cultural Geography* 3 (1): 39–59. New York: Bloomsbury.

New Directions in the Study of Prayer (NDSP). 2011. "New Directions in the Study of Prayer." New York: Social Sciences and Research Council. 1 September. https://www.ssrc.org/programs/component/religion-and-the-public-sphere/new-directions-in-the-study-of-prayer/.

Newitt, Mark. 2011. "The Role and Skills of a Chaplain." In *Being a Chaplain*, edited by Miranda Threfall-Holmes and Mark Newitt, 103–15. London: SPCK.

Nilsson, Kjell, Marcus Sangster, and Cecil C. Konijnendijk. 2011. "Forests, Trees and Human Health and Well-being: Introduction." In *Forests, Trees and Human Health*, edited by Kjell Nilsson, Marcus Sangster, Christos Gallis, Terry Hartig, Sjerp de Vries, Klaus Seeland, and Jasper Schipperijn, 1–19. New York: Springer.

Nongbri, Brent. 2013. *Before Religion: A History of a Modern Concept*. London: Yale University Press.

Norwood, Frances. 2006. "The Ambivalent Chaplain: Negotiating Structural and Ideological Difference on the Margins of Modern-Day Hospital Medicine." *Medical Anthropology* 25 (1): 1–29.

Office for National Statistics (ONS). 2012. *Religion in England and Wales 2011*. London: ONS. https://www.ons.gov.uk/peoplepopulationand community/culturalidentity/religion/articles/religioninenglandand wales2011/2012-12-11.

O'Kane, Caitlin. 2020. "Nurses and Doctors Stand on Hospital Rooftops to

Pray over Patients and Families." *CBS News*, 2 April. https://www.cbsnews
.com/news/coronavirus-doctors-nurses-praying-hospital-roofs-covid-19-
patients-families/.

Olsen, Bjørnar. 2003. "Material Culture after Text: Re-Membering Things."
Norwegian Archaeological Review 36 (2): 87–104.

Orchard, Helen C. 2000. *Hospital Chaplains: Modern, Dependable?* Sheffield:
Sheffield Academic.

Orsi, Robert. 1985. *The Madonna of 115th Street: Faith and Community in
Italian Harlem, 1880–1950.* New Haven, CT: Yale University Press.

– 2003. "Is the Study of Lived Religion Irrelevant to the World We Live in?
Special Presidential Plenary Address, Society for the Scientific Study of
Religion, Salt Lake City, 2 November 2002." *Journal for the Scientific Study
of Religion* 42: 169–74.

– 2005. *Between Heaven and Earth: The Religious Worlds People Make and the
Scholars Who Study Them.* Princeton: Princeton University Press.

Paradies, Yin, Mandy Truong, and Naomi Priest. 2014. "A Systematic Review
of the Extent and Measurement of Healthcare Provider Racism." *Journal
of General Internal Medicine* 29 (2): 364–87.

Pattison, Stephen. 2015. "Situating Chaplaincy in the United Kingdom: The
Acceptable Face of 'Religion'?" In *A Handbook of Chaplaincy Studies:
Understanding Spiritual Care in Public Places,* edited by Christopher Swift,
Mark Cobb, and Andrew Todd, 13–30. Farnham, UK: Ashgate.

Pesut, Barbara. 2015. "Critical Response to Palliative Case Studies: A Nurse's
Perspective." In *Spiritual Care in Practice: Case Studies in Healthcare Chaplaincy,* edited by George Fitchett and Steve Nolan, 272–81. London: Jessica Kingsley.

Pesut, Barbara, Marsha Fowler, Elizabeth J. Taylor, Sheryl Reimer-Kirkham,
and Richard Sawatzky. 2008. "Conceptualizing Spirituality and Religion
for Healthcare." *Journal of Clinical Nursing* 17 (21): 2803–10.

Pesut, Barbara, Sheryl Reimer-Kirkham, Richard Sawatzky, Gloria Wood-
land, and Perry Peverall. 2012. "Hospitable Hospitals in a Diverse Society:
From Chaplains to Spiritual Care Providers." *Journal of Religion and
Health* 51 (3): 825–36.

Pink, Sarah, and David Howes. 2010. "The Future of Sensory Anthropolo-
gy/The Anthropology of the Senses." *Social Anthropology* 18 (3): 331–3.

Powell, Kimberly. 2010. "Making Sense of Place: Mapping as a Multisensory
Research Method." *Qualitative Inquiry* 16 (7): 539–55.

Poynting, Scott, and Victoria Mason. 2007. "The Resistible Rise of Islamophobia: Anti-Muslim Racism in the UK and Australia before 11 September 2001." *Journal of Sociology* 43 (1): 61–86.

Pretty, Jules. 2004. "How Nature Contributes to Mental and Physical Health." *Spirituality and Health International* 5 (2): 68–78.

Putnam, Robert D. 2000. *Bowling Alone: The Collapse and Revival of American Community*. New York: Simon & Schuster.

Quinn, Barry. 2012. "The Project of Sense Making as Part of Illness: Exploring the Lived Experience of People with Cancer." PhD diss., King's College London.

– 2017. "Role of Nursing Leadership in Providing Compassionate Care." *Nursing Standard* 32 (16–19): 53–63. https://doi.org/10.7748/ns.2017.e11035.

Quinn, Sandra, and Supriya Kumar. 2014. "Health Inequalities and Infectious Disease Epidemics: A Challenge for Global Health Security." *Biosecurity and Bioterrorism*, 12 (5): 263–73.

Raffay, Julian, Emily Wood, and Andrew Todd. 2016. "Service User Views of Spiritual and Pastoral Care (Chaplaincy) in NHS Mental Health Services: A Co-Produced Constructivist Grounded Theory Investigation." *BMC Psychiatry* 16 (1): 200–11.

Reimer Kirkham, Sheryl. 2003. "The Politics of Belonging and Intercultural Health Care." *Western Journal of Nursing Research* 25 (7): 762–80.

Reimer-Kirkham, Sheryl, and Marie Cochrane. 2016. "Resistant, Reluctant or Responsible? The Negotiation of Religious and Cultural Plurality in Canadian Healthcare." In *Religion, Equalities and Inequalities*, edited by Dawn Llewellyn and Sonya Sharma, 65–76. London: Routledge.

Reimer-Kirkham, Sheryl, and Sonya Sharma. 2011. "Adding Religion to Gender, Race, and Class: Seeking New Insights on Intersectionality in Health Care Contexts." In *Health Inequities in Canada: Intersectional Frameworks and Practices*, edited by Olena Hankivsky, 112–27. Vancouver: UBC Press.

Reimer-Kirkham, Sheryl, Sonya Sharma, Sonya Grypma, Barbara Pesut, Richard Sawatzky, and Dorolen Wolfs. 2017. "'The Elephant on the Table': Religious and Ethnic Diversity in Home Health Services." *Journal of Religion and Health*. Advance online publication. doi.org/10.1007/s10943-017-0489-7.

Reimer-Kirkham, Sheryl, Sonya Sharma, Barb Pesut, Richard Sawatzky, Heather Meyerhoff, and Marie Cochrane. 2012. "Sacred Spaces in Public Places: Religious and Spiritual Plurality in Health Care." *Nursing Inquiry* 19 (3): 202–12.

Reimer-Kirkham, Sheryl, Sonya Sharma, and Brenda Corcoran Smith. 2019. "When Prayer Shows Up: The Social Relations of Prayer in Healthcare." Unpublished report. Langley, BC: Trinity Western University.

Reimer-Kirkham, Sheryl, Sonya Sharma, Brenda Smith, Kelly Schutt, and Kyla Janzen. 2018. "Expressions of Prayer in Residential Care Homes." *Journal of Health Care Chaplaincy* 24 (2): 67–85.

Riis, Ole, and Linda Woodhead. 2010. *A Sociology of Religious Emotion.* Oxford: Oxford University Press.

Rispler-Chaim, Vardit. 2006. *Disability in Islamic Law.* New York: Springer.

Robertson, Ruth, Lillie Wenzel, James Thompson, and Anna Charles. 2017. *Understanding NHS Financial Pressures: How Are They Affecting Patient Care?* King's Fund, 14 March. https://www.kingsfund.org.uk/publications /understanding-nhs-financial-pressures.

Robinson, Simon, Kevin Kendrick, and Alan Brown. 2003. *Spirituality and the Practice of Healthcare.* New York: Palgrave Macmillan.

Roychoudhuri, Onnesha. 2015. "'Nones,' Affiliation, and Prayer." *Reverberations: New Directions in the Study of Prayer.* 16 September. http://forums .ssrc.org/ndsp/2015/09/16/nones-affiliation-and-prayer/.

Rudgard, Olivia. 2017. "Christian Nurse Sacked for Offering to Pray with Patients Was Just Showing 'Compassion,' Tribunal Hears." *Telegraph,* 30 March. https://www.telegraph.co.uk/news/2017/03/30/christian-nurse-sacked-offering-pray-patients-just-showing-compassion/.

Saunders, Cicely. n.d. "Spiritual Pain." Originally published in *Hospital Chaplain*, March 1988, reproduced by permission & printed by A.G. Bishop & Sons: Orpington, Kent.

Savage, Mike. 2015. *Social Class in the 21st Century.* London: Penguin.

Schegloff, Emanuel A. 2007. *Sequence Organization in Interaction: A Primer in Conversation Analysis.* Cambridge: Cambridge University Press.

Schein, Edgar H. 2010. *Organizational Culture and Leadership.* San Francisco: John Wiley & Sons.

Selby, Jennifer, Amélie Barras, and Lori G. Beaman. 2018. *Beyond Accommodation: Everyday Narratives of Muslim Canadians.* Vancouver: UBC Press.

Selman, Lucy Ellen, Lisa Jane Brighton, Shane Sinclair, Ikali Karvinen, Richard Egan, Peter Speck, Richard A. Powell, et al. 2018. "Patients' and Caregivers' Needs, Experiences, Preferences and Research Priorities in Spiritual Care: A Focus Group Study across Nine Countries." *Palliative Medicine* 32 (1): 216–30.

Sharma, Sonya, and Mathew Guest. 2013. "Navigating Religion between University and Home: Christian Students' Experiences in English Universities." *Social & Cultural Geography* 14 (1): 59–79.

Sharma, Sonya, and Dawn Lewellyn. 2016. "Introduction: Religion, Equalities and Inequalities." In *Religion, Equalities and Inequalities*, edited by Dawn Llewellyn and Sonya Sharma, xvii–xxvii. London: Routledge.

Sharma, Sonya, and Sheryl Reimer-Kirkham. 2015. "Faith as Social Capital: Diasporic Women Negotiating Religion in Secularized Healthcare Services." *Women's Studies International Forum* 49 (March–April): 34–42.

Sharma, Sonya, Sheryl Reimer-Kirkham, and Marie Cochrane. 2009. "Practicing the Awareness of Embodiment in Qualitative Health Research: Methodological Reflections." *Qualitative Health Research* 19 (11): 1642–50.

– 2013. "Prayer as Transgression: Stories from Healthcare." In *Prayer in Religion and Spirituality*. Vol. 4 of *Annual Review of the Sociology of Religion*, edited by Guiseppe Giordan and Linda Woodhead, 189–204. Leiden, Netherlands: Brill.

Sheridan, Lorraine. 2006. "Islamophobia Pre– and Post–September 11th, 2001." *Journal of Interpersonal Violence* 21 (3): 317–36.

Smith, Pam. 2012. *The Emotional Labour of Nursing Revisited: Can Nurses Still Care?* 2nd ed. New York: Palgrave.

Socías, M. Eugenia, and Evan Wood. 2017. "Epidemic of Deaths from Fentanyl Overdose." *BMJ: British Medical Journal (Online)*: 358.

Soja, Edward. 2008. "Thirdspace: Toward a New Consciousness of Space and Spatiality." In *Communicating in the Third Space*, edited by Karin Ikas and Gerhard Wagner, 63–75. London: Routledge.

South Yorkshire NHS Workforce Development Confederation. 2003. *Caring for the Spirit: A Strategy for the Chaplaincy and Spiritual Care Workforce.* South Yorkshire: National Health Service. https://www.merseycare.nhs.uk/media/1856/caring-for-the-spirit.pdf.

Stammers, Trevor, and Stephen Bullivant. 2012. "Secularism." In *Oxford Textbook of Spirituality in Healthcare*, edited by Mark Cobb, Christina M. Puchalski, and Bruce Rumbold, 83–8. Oxford: Oxford University Press.

Staricoff, Rosalia, and Stephen Clift. 2011. *Arts and Music in Healthcare: An Overview of the Medical Literature: 2004–2011.* Chelsea and Westminster Health Charity, London. http://www.lahf.org.uk/sites/default/files/Chelsea%20and%20Westminster%20Literature%20Review%20Staricoff%20and%20Clift%20FINAL.pdf.

Statistics Canada. 2011. "National Household Survey." 23 November. http://www12.statcan.gc.ca/nhs-enm/2011/dp-pd/prof/index.cfm?Lang=E.

– 2017a. "Aboriginal Peoples in Canada: Key Results from the 2016 Census." 25 October. http://www.statcan.gc.ca/daily-quotidien/171025/dq171025a-eng.htm.

– 2017b. "2016 Census: Highlights from the Immigration and Ethnocultural Diversity in Canada Release." 19 January. https://www2.gov.bc.ca/gov/content/data/statistics/infoline/infoline-2017/17-135-2016-census-immigration-ethnocultural-diversity.

Stevenson, Deborah, and Liam Magee. 2017. "Art and Space: Creative Infra-structure and Cultural Capital in Sydney, Australia." *Journal of Sociology* 53 (4): 839–61.

Stokoe, Rodney. 1974. "Clinical Pastoral Education." *Nova Scotia Medical Bulletin*, February, 26–8.

Stringer, Martin. 2015. "Transcendence and Immanence in Public and Private Prayer." In *A Sociology of Prayer*, edited by Giuseppe Giordan and Linda Woodhead, 67–80. Farnham, UK: Ashgate.

Sullivan, Winnifred Fallers. 2014. *A Ministry of Presence: Chaplaincy, Spiritual Care, and the Law*. Chicago: University of Chicago Press.

Sun, Anna. 2016. "A Sociological Consideration of Prayer and Agency." *TDR: The Drama Review* 60 (4, T232, Winter): 118–29.

Sutton, David E. 2001. *Remembrance of Repasts: An Anthropology of Food and Memory*. New York: Berg.

Swift, Christopher. 2009. *Hospital Chaplaincy in the Twenty-First Century: The Crisis of Spiritual Care on the NHS*. Farnham, UK: Ashgate.

– 2015. "Health Care Chaplaincy." In *A Handbook of Chaplaincy Studies: Understanding Spiritual Care in Public Places*, edited by Christopher Swift, Mark Cobb, and Andrew Todd, 163–74. Farnham, UK: Ashgate.

Swift, Christopher, Mark Cobb, and Andrew Todd. 2015. *A Handbook of Chaplaincy Studies: Understanding Spiritual Care in Public Places*. Farnham, UK: Ashgate.

Swinton, John. 2001. *Spirituality and Mental Health Care: Rediscovering a "Forgotten" Dimension*. London: Jessica Kingsley.

– 2012. *Dementia: Living in the Memories of God*. Grand Rapids, MI: Eerdmans.

Tarlo, Emma. 2007. "Hijab in London: Metamorphosis, Resonance and Effects." *Journal of Material Culture* 12 (2): 131–56.

Taussig, Michael. 1998. "Transgression." In *Critical Terms for Religious Studies*, edited by Mark C. Taylor, 349–64. Chicago: University of Chicago Press.

Taves, Ann. 2009. *Religious Experience Reconsidered: A Building Block Approach to the Study of Religion and Other Special Things*. Princeton: Princeton University Press.

Taylor, Charles. 2007. *A Secular Age*. Cambridge, MA: Belknap of Harvard University Press.

Thin, Neil. 2009. "Why Anthropology Can Ill Afford to Ignore Well-being." In *Pursuits of Happiness: Well-being in Anthropological Perspective*, edited by Gordon Mathews and Carolina Izquierdo, 23–44. New York: Berghahn.

Threlfall-Holmes, Miranda, and Mark Newitt, eds. 2011a. *Being a Chaplain*. London: SPCK.

– 2011b. "Introduction." In Threlfall-Holmes and Newitt, *Being a Chaplain*, xiii–xix.

Todd, Andrew. 2015. "The Value of Spiritual Care: Negotiating Spaces and Practices for Spiritual Care in the Public Domain." In *Critical Care: Delivering Spiritual Care in Healthcare Contexts*, edited by Jonathan Pye, Peter Sedgwick, and Andrew Todd, 70–86. London: Jessica Kingsley.

Todd, Douglas. 2010. "Do Hospital Chaplains Deserve Public Funding?" *Vancouver Sun*, 11 January. http://vancouversun.com/news/staff-blogs /update-do-hospital-chaplains-deserve-public-funding.

– 2013. "Religions Work Together on Richmond's Highway to Heaven." *Vancouver Sun*, 9 August. http://www.vancouversun.com/life/Douglas +Todd+Religions+work+together+Richmond+Highway+Heaven/8771141/ story.html.

Tronto, Joan C. 1994. *Moral Boundaries: A Political Argument for an Ethic of Care*. London: Routledge.

Truth and Reconciliation Commission of Canada (TRC). 2015. *Honouring the Truth, Reconciling for the Future: Summary of the Final Report of the Truth and Reconciliation Commission of Canada*. Winnipeg, MB: Truth and Reconciliation Commission of Canada, 31 May. http://publications.gc.ca /site/eng/9.800288/publication.html.

Turner, Victor. (1969) 2017. *The Ritual Process: Structure and Anti-Structure*. London: Routledge.

– 1974. *The Ritual Process: Structure and Anti-Structure*. Hardmonsdworth, Middlesex: Penguin.

Tweed, Thomas. 2006. *Crossing and Dwelling: A Theory of Religion*. Cambridge, MA: Harvard University Press.

UK Board of Healthcare Chaplaincy (UKBHC). 2020. "Welcome to the UK Board of Healthcare Chaplaincy." https://www.ukbhc.org.uk/.

Ungerson, Clare. 1990. "The Language of Care: Crossing the Boundaries." Chapter 1 in *Gender and Caring: Work and Welfare in Britain and Scandinavia*. London: Harvester Wheatsheaf.

VandeCreek, Larry, and Laurel Burton. 2001. "A White Paper. Professional Chaplaincy: Its Role and Importance in Healthcare." *Journal of Pastoral Care & Counseling* 55 (1): 81–97.

van den Berg, Agnes E. 2005. *Health Impacts of Healing Environments: A Review of Evidence for Benefits of Nature, Daylight, Fresh Air, and Quiet in Healthcare Settings*. Groningen, Netherlands: Foundation 200 Years, University Hospital Groningen.

van der Riet, Pamela, Chaweewan Jitsacorn, Piyatida Junlapeeya, Erin Thursby, and Peter Thursby. 2017. "Family Members' Experiences of a 'Fairy Garden' Healing Haven Garden for Sick Children." *Collegian: The Australian Journal for Nursing Practice, Scholarship and Research* 24 (2): 165–73.

van der Veer, Peter. 2016. "Introduction." Special Issue: Prayer and Politics. *Journal of Religious and Political Practice* 2 (1): 1–5.

van Gennep, Arnold. 1960. *The Rites of Passage*. Chicago: University of Chicago Press.

Vásquez, Manuel, and Kim Knott. 2014. "Three Dimensions of Religious Place Making in Diaspora." *Global Networks* 14 (3): 326–47.

Vertovec, Steven. 2007. "Super-Diversity and Its Implications." *Ethnic and Racial Studies* 30 (6): 1024–54.

Vigh, Henry. 2008. "Crisis and Chronicity: Anthropological Perspectives on Continuous Conflict and Decline." *Ethnos* 73 (1): 5–24.

Vincett, Giselle, Sonya Sharma, and Kristin Aune. 2008. "Introduction: Women, Religion and Secularization in the West: One Size Does Not Fit All." In *Women and Religion in the West: Challenging Secularization*, edited by Kristin Aune, Sonya Sharma, and Giselle Vincett, 1–22. Aldershot, UK: Ashgate.

Wall, Jeff. 1990. *The Pine on the Corner*. Vancouver, BC: Collection of the Vancouver Art Gallery.

Weber, Beverly M. 2015. "Gender, Race, Religion, Faith? Rethinking Intersectionality in German Feminisms." *European Journal of Women's Studies* 22 (1): 22–36.

Weber, Samuel R., and Kenneth Pargament I. 2014. "The Role of Religion and Spirituality in Mental Health." *Current Opinion in Psychiatry* 27 (5): 358–63.

Wellcome Trust. 2017. *A Museum of Nature Exhibition*. https://wellcomecollection.org/exhibitions/museum-modern-nature.

Weller, Paul, Tristram Hooley, and Nicki Moore. 2011. *Religion and Belief in Higher Education: The Experiences of Staff and Students*. London: London Equality Challenge Unit.

Werbner, Pnina. 2010. "Religious Identity." In *The Sage Handbook of Identities*, edited by Margaret Wetherell and Chandra Talpade Mohanty, 233–57. London: Sage.

Wilkins, Amy C. 2008. *Wannabes, Goths, and Christians: The Boundaries of Sex, Style, and Status*. Chicago: University of Chicago Press.

Wilkins-Laflamme, Sarah. 2017a. *The Religious, Spiritual, Secular and Social Landscapes of the Pacific Northwest – Part 1*. UWSpace. https://uwspace.uwaterloo.ca/handle/10012/12218.

– 2017b. "Religious-Secular Polarization Compared: The Cases of Quebec and British Columbia." *Studies in Religion / Sciences Religieuses* 42 (2): 166–85.

Wilson, Ceri, Hilary Bungay, Carol Munn-Giddings, and Melanie Boyce. 2016. "Healthcare Professionals' Perceptions of the Value and Impact of the Arts in Healthcare Settings: A Critical Review of the Literature." *International Journal of Nursing Studies* 56 (April): 90–101.

Wilson, Kathleen. 2003. "Therapeutic Landscapes and First Nations Peoples: An Exploration of Culture, Health and Place." *Health & Place* 9 (2): 83–93.

Winchester, Margaret, and Janet McGrath. 2017. "Therapeutic Landscapes." *Medicine Anthropology Theory* 4 (1): i–x.

Woodhead, Linda. 2012. "Introduction." In *Religion and Change in Modern Britain*, edited by Linda Woodhead and Rebecca Catto, 1–33. London: Routledge.

– 2015a. "Chaplaincy and the Future of Religion." In *A Handbook of Chaplaincy Studies: Understanding Spiritual Care in Public Places*, edited by Christopher Swift, Andrew Todd, and Mark Cobb, xvii–xxii. Farnham, UK: Ashgate.

– 2015b. "Conclusion: Prayer as Changing the Subject." In *A Sociology of Prayer*, edited by Guiseppe Giordan and Linda Woodhead, 213–30. Farnham, UK: Ashgate.

– 2016. "The Rise of 'No Religion' in Britain: The Emergence of a New Cultural Majority." *Journal of the British Academy* 4: 245–61.

– 2017. "2016 Paul Hanly Furfey Lecture. The Rise of 'No Religion': Towards an Explanation." *Sociology of Religion: A Quarterly Review* 78 (3): 247–62.

World Health Organization. n.d. "WHO Definition of Palliative Care." http://www.who.int/cancer/palliative/definition/en/.

Wuthnow, Robert. 2008. "Prayer, Cognition, and Culture." *Poetics* 36 (5–6): 333–7.

Yip, Andrew K-T. 2000. "Leaving the Church to Keep My Faith: The Lived Experiences of Non-Heterosexual Christians." In *Joining and Leaving Religion: Research Perspectives*, edited by Leslie J. Francis and Yaacov J. Katz, 129–46. Leominster: Gracewing.

– 2003. "Sexuality and the Church." *Sexualities* 6 (1): 60–4.

Ze'ev, Maghen. 2005. *Virtues of the Flesh: Passion and Purity in Early Islamic Jurisprudence*. Leiden, Netherlands: Brill.

Zimonjic, Peter. 2020 "Keeping the Faith during the COVID-19 Pandemic – by Praying at Home and Staying Connected Online." *Vancouver Sun*, 30

March. https://www.cbc.ca/news/politics/pandemic-religion-islam-jewish-christian-1.5515588.

Zock, Hetty. 2008. "The Split Professional Identity of the Chaplain as a Spiritual Caregiver in Contemporary Dutch Health Care: Are There Implications for the United States?" *Journal of Pastoral Care and Counseling* 62: 137–9.

Contributors

LORI G. BEAMAN, PhD, is Canada Research Chair in Religious Diversity and Social Change, professor at the University of Ottawa, and principal investigator of the Nonreligion and a Complex Future Project (https://nonreligionproject.ca/). Publications include *Deep Equality in an Era of Religious Diversity* (Oxford University Press, 2017). She received the 2017 SSHRC Insight Award and holds an honorary doctorate from Uppsala University.

CHRISTINA BEARDSLEY, PhD, is a Church of England priest and retired healthcare chaplain, and a visiting scholar within the Centre for Human Flourishing at Sarum College, Salisbury, England. Her publications include articles on spirituality and chaplaincy, co-authored books about transgender people's spiritual care, and the biography *Unutterable Love: The Passionate Life & Preaching of FW Robertson* (Lutterworth, 2009).

PAUL BRAMADAT, PhD, is professor and director of the Centre for Studies in Religion and Society at the University of Victoria. Recent publications include *Public Health in the Age of Anxiety* (University of Toronto Press, 2017). He is principal investigator of a SSHRC-funded project on religion, irreligion, and secularity in the Pacific Northwest of North America.

RACHEL BROWN, PhD, is the Religious Studies Teaching Fellow at the Centre for Studies in Religion and Society, University of Victoria. She has published on lived religion, religion and migration, and foodways, and is completing a book, entitled *Consuming Identity*. As a collaborator on a SSHRC-funded project, her research is on the experience of religious minorities in the Pacific Northwest.

MELANIA CALESTANI, PhD, is lecturer at Kingston and St George's, University of London. She has been involved in projects on well-being, religion, and spirituality, and published on decision-making and patient-centred care. Publications include *An Anthropological Journey into Well-Being: Insights from Bolivia* (Springer, 2013), and *Youth on Religion: The Development, Negotiation and Impact of Faith and Non-Faith Identity* (Routledge, 2014).

SYLVIA COLLINS-MAYO, PhD, is associate professor in sociology of religion and head of Department of Criminology and Sociology at Kingston University London. Her work has focused on young people's faith and public engagement with prayer. She is co-author of *The Faith of Generation Y* (Church House Publishing, 2010) and *Religion and Youth* (Ashgate, 2010).

BRENDA CORCORAN SMITH, MSN, is a research associate in the School of Nursing at Trinity Western University and a practicing occupational health nurse. She was project coordinator for *Prayer as Transgression? Exploring Accommodation of And Resistance to Prayer in Public Spaces.* Recent publications include (as co-author) journal article "Expressions of Prayer in Residential Care Homes."

CHRISTOPHER E. DE BONO, MDiv, PhD, is the vice president of Mission, People and Ethics for Providence Health Care in Vancouver, British Columbia, Canada. A Roman Catholic pastoral theologian, a clinical and organizational ethicist, and a certified Spiritual Care chaplain, his research interests include the integration of spirituality/religion in clinical care.

BARRY QUINN, PhD, has held numerous senior nursing leadership roles within the NHS in London and is currently a senior lecturer in nursing and philosophical studies at Queen's University Belfast. He chairs two European multi-professional cancer and palliative care working groups. He is consultant editor for *Nursing Management*, a leading nursing journal, and has published extensively on the human component of healthcare and cancer-related topics.

SHERYL REIMER-KIRKHAM, PhD, is dean and professor of nursing, Trinity Western University. Her research focuses on plurality, equity, and human rights in healthcare, focusing on the intersections of spirituality, race, class, and gender. She has published extensively on these topics and is co-editor of *Religion, Religious Ethics, and Nursing* (Springer, 2012). Her scholarship has been recognized with numerous awards.

SONYA SHARMA, PhD, is associate professor in sociology at Kingston University London. She has researched on religion and spirituality in healthcare, religion and intimacy between sisters and the work of women healthcare chaplains. She has published on these areas and is co-editor of *Women and Religion in the West: Challenging Secularization* (Ashgate, 2008) and *Religion, Equalities and Inequalities* (Routledge, 2016).

ANDREW TODD, PhD, is senior lecturer and director of the Professional Doctorate in Practical Theology at Anglia Ruskin University and the Cambridge Theological Federation. He has led a number of funded research projects on chaplaincy and religion, publishing widely in this field, including: C. Swift, M. Cobb, and A. Todd, eds, *A Handbook of Chaplaincy Studies* (Ashgate, 2015).

Index